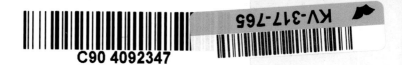

PRAISE FOR **THE YOGA EFFECT**

"*The Yoga Effect* offers a window into how ancient practices affect our minds and moods. It is a fine example of the collaboration between yoga teachers and brain researchers exploring the use of yoga in mental health treatment."

—Patricia L. Gerbarg, MD, assistant professor in clinical psychiatry, New York Medical College, and coauthor of *The Healing Power of the Breath*

"Readers will find an excellent review of the basics of yoga theory and practice in addition to well-presented instructions on a wide range of specific yoga practices that are likely to improve mental health and well-being. The research described in *The Yoga Effect* has been a meaningful contribution to the field."

—Sat Bir Singh Khalsa, PhD, assistant professor of medicine, Harvard Medical School, and chief editor of *The Principles and Practice of Yoga in Health Care*

"In an inspirational collaboration, yoga teacher Liz Owen, writer Holly Rossi, and medical researcher Chris Streeter forge new ground for how yoga can be researched and validated within the western medical framework without devaluing their personal experiences with yoga as a healing mechanism. By making our best efforts to combine the best of both worlds, like these authors, we have an opportunity to make some real progress."

—David Emerson, director of The Center for Trauma and Embodiment at JRI, author of *Trauma-Sensitive Yoga in Therapy*, and coauthor of *Overcoming Trauma through Yoga*

THE YOGA EFFECT

THE
YOGA
EFFECT

A PROVEN PROGRAM
FOR DEPRESSION AND ANXIETY

LIZ OWEN & HOLLY LEBOWITZ ROSSI
with Chris C. Streeter, MD

Photography by Tracy Rodriguez

First published in the United States in 2019 by Da Capo Lifelong Books, Hachette Book Group
Da Capo Lifelong Books is an imprint of Perseus Books, LLC, a subsidiary of Hachette Book Group, Inc.
1290 Avenue of the Americas, New York, NY 10104

This edition published in Great Britain in 2019 by Orion Spring
an imprint of The Orion Publishing Group Ltd
Carmelite House, 50 Victoria Embankment
London EC4Y 0DZ

An Hachette UK Company

1 3 5 7 9 10 8 6 4 2

A CIP catalogue record for this book is
available from the British Library.

ISBN (Trade Paperback) 9781409195344
ISBN (eBook) 9781409195351

Printed and bound in Great Britain by Clays Ltd, Elcograf, S.p.A

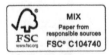

MIX
Paper from
responsible sources
FSC
www.fsc.org   FSC® C104740

www.orionbooks.co.uk

ORION
SPRING

*To all my students and teachers, with great
gratitude for your gifts—LO*

*For my parents, the keepers of my history and
my eternal* consiglieres—HLR

NOTE TO THE READER

This book is not intended as a substitute for medical advice or treatment. Before beginning any yoga or other exercise program, please consult a physician.

The yoga practices in this book, and in the studies that the book is based on, were created to be as accessible to as many people as possible, so that anyone living with depression or anxiety may find yoga to be a meaningful tool on a healing journey. The Iyengar style of yoga, because of its comprehensive teacher training protocols and its use of props and pose modifications, is the basis of the yoga in both the studies and the book.

In this time of much-needed and appropriate scrutiny of human interactions within organizations and society, we unequivocally state our support for victims and survivors of any form of abuse, both within and outside of the yoga community. Our mission is to promote a sense of safety and encourage self-exploration, recovery, restoration, and self-actualization for all who open this book, and indeed, for all who come to yoga for help.

If you need emotional help, please contact a mental health professional in your area. If you are in crisis, please call the National Suicide Prevention Lifeline (1-800-273-8255) or 911.

The names and identifying details of individuals who participated in scientific research described in this book have been changed to protect their privacy.

CONTENTS

FOREWORD

In ninth grade, I took my first yoga class, and I have been intrigued by the mind-body relationship ever since—so much so that the opening sentence in my medical school application was, "I want to study the mind, body, soul interface." This led to a path that included training in neurology, behavioral neurology, and psychiatry in the pursuit of understanding how yoga practices affect how we feel and how yoga might be useful in treating mental illness, specifically depression.

I have long been interested in what I call the "round-peg-square-hole dilemma" of trying to understand yoga philosophy through the lens of Western science, because if both disciplines are correct, they should not be in conflict. I am delighted that Liz Owen, a gifted yoga instructor and my longtime collaborator, along with her writing partner Holly Lebowitz Rossi, have taken the opportunity to meld Western scientific research and yoga philosophy and practice into a book that people can use to understand and improve the symptoms of depression and anxiety.

Over the course of three scientific studies I've collaborated on with Liz, we developed a protocol that focused on the yoga postures thought to be beneficial for improving the symptoms of depression. Our first study's participants had no diagnosis of depression, while the second study involved people with Major Depressive Disorder and added a breathing exercise to the yoga postures. Our third study is a randomized, controlled trial comparing walking to yoga as a treatment for depression. All of these studies used magnetic resonance imaging (MRI) technology to measure chemical changes in the brain before and after the yoga practice. Our approach has allowed us to observe improvement in mood in a healthy population and improvement of depressive and anxious symptoms in individuals diagnosed with depression. This book provides a practical manual that is based on the program Liz and I developed.

Through my collaboration with Liz, over the course of more than a decade, I had the privilege and honor of also collaborating with many wonderful and skilled yoga instructors, including Patricia Walden, an internationally recognized expert in the teaching of the Iyengar method of yoga, who has long advocated for using yoga to treat depression.

Although it is my observation that the different schools of yoga are more similar than different, I chose the Iyengar method for the studies. Iyengar yoga instructors are required to undergo a rigorous training and certification process, which leaves them highly skilled in how to modify the postures to meet the ability of each student, frequently using props such as blankets and blocks. This allows the protocol Liz and I developed to be accessible to a broad audience, amplifying the potential for its widespread use and benefit.

Yoga is not a substitute for antidepressant medications, but the addition of a yoga practice to a treatment plan incorporating antidepressants can enhance and expand your toolkit of treatments. People in the United States are practicing yoga in greater and greater numbers, and there is considerable evidence that they use it to treat medical problems as well as to foster overall wellness. I look forward to working on more multidisciplinary studies that will add to the current body of evidence on how to integrate yoga into medical treatment.

I hope that you find this book as accessible and helpful as I did. It melds the findings of Western science and yoga philosophy in a way that is both useful as a guide to practice and illuminating in terms of understanding why a yoga practice can foster an emotionally healthy lifestyle.

Chris C. Streeter, MD
Boston, Massachusetts

To know yourself as the Being underneath the thinker, the stillness underneath the mental noise, the love and joy underneath the pain, is freedom, salvation, enlightenment.

—Eckhart Tolle, The Power of Now

PREFACE

How to Use This Book

Living with depression and anxiety is challenging enough—this book is meant to help ease your symptoms, not add to your mental load. To this end, I have organized the book in a way I hope is accessible, interesting, and inspiring. Before you turn to Chapter 1, I want to lay out the book's structure so you can get the greatest benefit from it.

First, you will note that there are two authors' names on the cover, but to make your reading experience easier, we have chosen to use a collective "I" pronoun throughout the book.

As you read, you'll note that the first four chapters are grouped under the heading, "Science and Yoga for Emotional Health." In Chapter 1, I review the science that makes yoga a powerful tool in the journey toward emotional wellness—something Amy Weintraub, in her book *Yoga for Depression*, calls "preventative and positive medicine."[1]

In Chapters 2 and 3, I explore the philosophical concepts that undergird our work together, from ancient ideas about energy and emotion to the relationship between your physical and mental bodies. In Chapter 4, you will prepare for a series of yoga practices that directly address each of five emotional goals—centeredness, empowerment, energy, calm, and balance. Then you will be ready to step onto your mat and explore each of these attributes in depth.

The second section of the book, "Yoga Practices for Depression and Anxiety," contains what I call the five "practice chapters," each of which aligns with one of the emotional attributes you were introduced to in Chapter 4. Each chapter presents a sequence of yoga poses and breathing exercises that will help you on your journey toward emotional wholeness. I offer modifications and tips for how to practice poses in complete comfort throughout—you should not abide pain as you practice. You can expect each practice to take you between twenty and forty-five minutes, depending on your pace, energy level, and general comfort.

While I recommend you read the book from cover to cover, I understand that you might be eager to get started with your practice as soon as possible. If that's the case, please be sure to read Chapter 4 first so you are physically and emotionally prepared for the journey ahead. Alternatively, you might wish to read Chapters 1–3 separately from the practice chapters, so you can absorb the scientific and philosophical information they contain.

Each practice chapter features "Three Questions to Prepare You for Practice." These questions are meant to plant seeds for thought, reflection, and insight that might change and develop as you move through each pose. It can be very helpful to take a moment to consider the questions at the beginning of the chapter. After you have finished your practice, we will ask you to reflect again. You might have some true aha moments as your yoga practice influences your thoughts and feelings.

Throughout the book, you will notice sidebars, which I've called "A Deeper Exploration" because they give me the opportunity to share extra tidbits I think might illuminate your journey. As you move through the practice chapters, feel free to integrate the additional information into your understanding of each emotional attribute—or skip them and come back to them once you are comfortable and familiar with the main material.

I have approached this book with understanding, empathy, and great respect for the challenges that come with the daily experience of depression, anxiety, or both. The many symptoms of depression and anxiety, or the side effects of medication, might have stopped you from attempting to develop a yoga practice before now. It is my deep hope that in these pages you can find your way into yoga—at your own pace, in whatever ways suit your needs in the moment—and that your practice becomes a source of support and peace in your life.

SCIENCE AND YOGA FOR
EMOTIONAL HEALTH

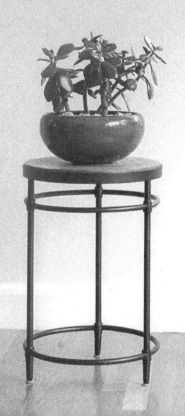

CHAPTER I

THE JOURNEY TOWARD BECOMING WHOLE AGAIN

Mahatma Gandhi once said, "The future depends on what we do in the present."[1] If you are reading these words in the midst of a struggle with depression or anxiety, you have taken a brave and important step in this present moment, one that I earnestly believe will illuminate a path toward a more positive future.

What is this great act of courage? It's nothing more complicated than the decision you made to pick up this book.

Now, let's not get ahead of ourselves. As much as I wish it were, this book isn't a magic wand that can permanently vaporize the weight of depression or tamp down the spiral of anxiety. No single book can do that, nor can any one therapy session, prescription, guided meditation, or yoga pose.

Why, then, is opening this book a healing act? How can it help you along the road back to wholeness from the stuck, uncomfortable place of depression and anxiety?

I believe the answer to that question lies in those words spoken by Gandhi. What stands out to me most in his statement is how vast, complex, and multifaceted those two categories of time—"the present" and "the future"—actually are. No single choice, no single action gets us from here to there. Instead, each of the myriad decisions we make in the here and now shapes the future we hope to see. It is my hope and intention that this book might become one healing choice among many that can set you on a path toward a better tomorrow.

All human beings struggle with difficult emotions at some point in their lives, whether they have a mental health diagnosis or not. And though so-called negative emotions like fear, sadness, and anger are often dismissed and discouraged in modern culture, those emotions serve a purpose in the big picture of our inner lives.

But those feelings aren't serving their purpose if they feel unmanageable to you on a regular basis. According to the National Institutes of Health, 21 percent of American adults—that's more than one in five—experience a mood disorder at some point in their lives.[2] Your journey toward wholeness starts with an honest appraisal of what most challenges you here, now, in the present moment.

Which is where yoga comes in.

YOGA AS A TOOL OF THE MIND

Yoga, like any system of thought, belief, and action, has a central set of teachings that define its purpose and perspective. One of these writings, compiled around the year 400 CE, is called *The Yoga Sutras of Patañjali*, and it describes the what, how, and why of the practice we understand today as yoga.

Let's consider this collection by the numbers. There are 196 sutras. Three have to do with physical poses; five more describe breath work and its effects.[3] The remaining 188 teachings focus on a single purpose—how to understand the mind and the human experience of consciousness, with a goal of becoming free from suffering.[4]

How remarkable that virtually the entire foundation of yoga is built around the philosophy of a disciplined mind, one that is organized, focused, present, reflective, discerning, and tranquil.

Given how fundamentally the practice is rooted in the mind-body relationship, it's no wonder that for decades, scientists have been investigating the connection between yoga and mental health. Literally hundreds of studies have examined yoga practice and inquired about its effectiveness, especially those "how" and "why" questions Patañjali considered in the sutras.

As you keep reading, let each passing page anchor Gandhi's suggestion more deeply in your mind. None of us can know or control the future, but by choosing to invest our time in healing actions again and again, here and now, in the present moment, we can take steady steps toward wellness, toward wholeness—toward our fully authentic selves.

WHAT MAKES THIS BOOK "EVIDENCE-BASED"

Throughout my thirty years teaching yoga, I have seen it change the lives of my students in profound and permanent ways. I have seen pain resolve into peace. I have seen inflexibility evolve into elasticity. I have seen people open their eyes to their own bodies, seeing themselves in new, transformative ways. I have taught college students; expectant mothers; those living with chronic fatigue syndrome, scoliosis, and multiple sclerosis; and people struggling with chronic challenges ranging from breathing disorders to weight management to pain to depression and anxiety.

When I met Dr. Chris Streeter, an associate professor of psychiatry and neurology at Boston University School of Medicine in 2006, I got an opportunity to dive more deeply into what I already understood about how profoundly yoga practice affects people, however life has challenged them.

Dr. Streeter invited me to work with her on a series of scientific studies about how yoga impacts mental health. Over the years since, I have learned more about those "how" and "why" insights that have captivated philosophers and scientists alike over the centuries.

When I partnered with Dr. Streeter, she had already completed some research on this topic, including a promising pilot study that found experienced yoga practitioners had an increase in a brain chemical called gamma aminobutyric acid (if attempting to pronounce that is making your heart pound, fear not: it is also referred to with the simple acronym GABA) after just an hour of practicing yoga postures.[5] GABA is a neurotransmitter, a chemical messenger that delivers information from one area of your brain to another. It's known as an "inhibitory neurotransmitter," meaning that when GABA attaches to receptors in the brain, it makes brain cells, called neurons, less likely to release other chemicals into your system or take another action.[6] If you have taken or considered antidepressant medications, you might note that a popular class of drugs is called selective serotonin reuptake inhibitors. SSRIs also work in an inhibitory way, slowing the rate at which serotonin—another neurotransmitter we need to manage our moods—is reabsorbed into the brain.[7]

GABA has been the focus of Dr. Streeter's subsequent research, as she's investigated how GABA affects mental health and how yoga impacts GABA levels. Over the course of three separate studies, my role was to lead a team of yoga teachers, under the mentorship of the noted Iyengar yoga teacher Patricia Walden, in creating a manual of the precise sequences of yoga poses and breath work that participants would undertake during their twelve weeks of yoga practice.

As you will soon learn, these studies produced very positive results, making groundbreaking observations about the association between yoga practice and improved mental health. The book you are holding in your hands is based on the practices our study participants did on their journeys toward wellness.

A Deeper Exploration: Why Iyengar Yoga Was Right for Our Research

By the time I met Dr. Streeter in 2006, it had been my good fortune to have studied Iyengar yoga for almost twenty years with one of its preeminent teachers, Patricia Walden. The Iyengar method is commonly referred to as a physical alignment–based yoga system. B. K. S. Iyengar (1918–2014) pioneered the use of yoga props and pose modifications to help people with physical limitations experience the benefits of yoga. In addition, he developed therapeutic applications of classical yoga to help manage many physical and mental conditions, depression and anxiety among them.[8]

Through Walden's and Iyengar's depth of knowledge, I learned so much more than how to achieve physical and energetic alignments and use props appropriately. I also learned the subtleties of working with the physical body to help shift mental and emotional energy toward a state of health and well-being. I learned techniques and tools that helped students feel better overall because they discovered a sense of inner peace.

Walden found that Iyengar yoga helped her with her own clinical depression.[9] She took a keen personal interest in Dr. Streeter's research, which uses the Iyengar method because its consistent and specific technique is easy to replicate in a scientific context. Walden eventually took on the role of mentoring our team as we developed and taught yoga sequences to the participants in the studies.

YOGA SCIENCE: THE BIGGER PICTURE

Scientists have been interested in yoga for more than a century.[10] But it's only since the 1970s that more funding and widespread interest in the West has led to a substantial body of research exploring the science of how yoga actually works.

The question of whether and how yoga affects emotional well-being has been a much-studied topic; the studies discussed in this book were funded by the National Institutes of Health's National Center for Complementary and Integrative Health and have been published in the peer-reviewed scientific publication the *Journal of Alternative and Complementary Medicine*. If you are reading this book because you are suffering from depression, anxiety, or both, know that a significant number of the hundreds of studies on yoga and mental health have yielded promising or positive results.

Good science is rooted in inquisitiveness, the willingness to pursue a question knowing its answer will lead to further inquiries to explore. Researchers have examined the connection between yoga and mental health around a number of questions, including the effects of different breathing speeds on stress, anxiety, and depression, the effects of yoga on post-traumatic stress disorder (PTSD), how yoga affects younger and older practitioners' mental health differently, and so much more.[11] New research is continuing to emerge even as I write these words.

THE BRAIN SCIENCE BEHIND OUR RESEARCH

So what has research contributed to the broader body of knowledge on yoga and mental health? In a nutshell . . . a lot. Its contribution zooms in from the broad concept of "the mind," which so occupied Patañjali, and instead focuses on arguably the most complex organ in the human body—the brain.

Dr. Streeter's research began with the observation that depression, anxiety, and epilepsy were all treated with drugs that increased the activity of what scientists call "the GABA system"—and the simultaneous observation that symptoms decreased in all three disorders during a yoga intervention. She wondered whether a yoga session might be associated with increased GABA levels and improved mood in healthy subjects. The premise was that low GABA levels were associated with lower mood and heightened anxiety. Some studies refer to GABA as a "natural antidepressant" because the more of it you have, the less depressive or anxious your moods are likely to be.[12]

To delve more deeply into the important role of GABA in mental health, Dr. Streeter set out to study this question: how, if at all, is the practice of yoga postures associated with changes in GABA levels?

Study I: For Emotional Health, How Does Yoga Compare with Walking?

Our first study together was published in 2010.[13] Thirty-four study participants were divided into two groups—nineteen completed a twelve-week program of twice-weekly yoga classes, while fifteen others did a twelve-week walking program. None of the participants was experienced in yoga, and none had a mental health diagnosis such as Major Depressive Disorder or Generalized Anxiety Disorder.

Dr. Streeter and her scientific team measured the participants' moods using two techniques. One was a pair of self-reported tests: the Exercise-Induced Feeling Inventory (EFI) and the State-Trait Anxiety Inventory (STAI).[14] The other was a brain scan called magnetic resonance spectroscopy, or MR spectroscopy (MRS). This scan is conducted on the same machine as an MRI, but it supplements the information provided by MRI scans with an additional measure of chemical levels in particular regions of the brain. Our MRS scans were designed to measure GABA levels in the thalamus, the region of the brain that has a high concentration of GABA and is connected to the circuits that modulate emotions and thoughts throughout the central nervous system.[15]

Both the walkers and the yoga practitioners completed the self-reported tests four times throughout the twelve weeks. They underwent the scans three times— once before the first session of either yoga or walking, and twice more after the twelve-week intervention was complete. Both those scans were done on the same day—once before and once after a final session of either yoga or walking.

The results of the study were extremely positive. Both groups experienced improvements in mood, but the yoga group had a greater boost—and only the yoga group showed an increase in GABA levels. This suggested that mood improvement is associated with increased GABA levels—and that yoga practice is associated with this positive correlation.[16]

Armed with this solid finding, but not yet able to assert proof that changes in GABA levels improve mood, Dr. Streeter decided it was time to ask more questions.

A Deeper Exploration: Your Autonomic Nervous System[17]

Brain science is a deeply complex field, and it's not my intention to bring you up to speed on all of its particulars. But there is a bit of this science that's so fundamental to how we function from moment to moment that I feel it is worth explaining in a chart you can reference whenever it's helpful to you. Think of this as an introduction to the two main components of your autonomic nervous system (ANS): the sympathetic nervous system (SNS) and the parasympathetic nervous system (PNS). These systems of basic, involuntary brain activities contribute to the modulation of your thoughts, feelings, and actions every moment of your life.

SYMPATHETIC NERVOUS SYSTEM (SNS)	PARASYMPATHETIC NERVOUS SYSTEM (PNS)
Prepares your body for physical and mental activity	Is responsible for bodily functions when you are at rest
Increases heart rate and raises blood pressure	Slows heart rate and lowers blood pressure
Inhibits digestion	Stimulates digestion
Stimulates the release of stress hormones like adrenaline, cortisol, and norepinephrine	Governs the "social engagement system" of your brain, including facial expressions and vocalization
Triggers the "fight-or-flight" response	Triggers the "relaxation response," also called the "rest and digest" and "tend and befriend" responses

These two systems complement each other: The SNS is responsible for fight-or-flight feelings and actions, while the PNS is responsible for rest, renewal, and social engagement.[18] I'm sure you can easily remember an experience in which you felt stressed—your breath probably quickened and your heart raced as your SNS activated. Now recall an instance in which you felt happy, perhaps when you were in a place where you felt safe and

(continues)

(continued)

relaxed—your breath and heart rate likely slowed as your PNS took over. Note the role of your breath in your autonomic nervous system's functioning. In fact, it subtly activates each time you breathe—the SNS when you inhale, and the PNS when you exhale.

Increased SNS activation is appropriate during times of extreme stress, when stress hormones increase as you navigate the crisis. But after the acute stress has passed, your heart rate needs to come back down to a resting, PNS-dominant state. When that doesn't happen, your nervous system remains in a state of heightened vigilance and overactivity, stuck in its SNS-dominant state. The cost of that excessive SNS activity could include depression, anxiety, PTSD, and chronic pain.[19]

In a bit, you'll learn more about a helpful way to think about the PNS, called the polyvagal theory. But for now, take a few slow, deep breaths and visualize the two halves of your autonomic nervous system working together to reflect your current mood. Are you stressed? Relaxed? Somewhere in between? Meet yourself right where you are on your journey toward wholeness.

Study 2: Is More Better When It Comes to Yoga?

Back in 2007, Dr. Streeter had conducted a pilot study using experienced yoga practitioners compared to participants, called the "control group" in science parlance, who did not do yoga.[20] It was the first time she had probed the idea that yoga practice might correlate with increased GABA levels, though that study did not measure any changes in mood during yoga practice. As we would later find in our work together, she noted an increase in GABA levels among the yoga practitioners after sixty minutes of yoga postures, while the control group read for sixty minutes and experienced no measurable change in GABA levels.

The change in GABA levels in that pilot study was extraordinary—the experienced yoga practitioners showed a 34 percent GABA increase in the thalamus.[21] Three years later, we found a still significant but less marked 13 percent increase in the thalami of participants who were beginners to yoga before the twelve-week program.

So the next question emerged—when it came to yoga practice, was more time on the mat better for mental health?

The technical term for our next study (published in 2017) was "dosing study," meaning that the yoga was practiced in "doses" of either two or three ninety-minute

sessions per week, plus either three or four thirty-minute weekly homework assign-
ments, respectively.[22] In addition to the yoga sequences, we added a meditative
breath practice called "Coherent Breathing" to each class session and homework
assignment. You'll learn more about Coherent Breathing later, in Chapter 4; it is
a technique in which inhales and exhales are practiced in an even rhythm, with
a goal of slowing breath to a rate of between three and one-half to six breaths per
minute, depending on the individual. This technique is described in detail in *The
Healing Power of the Breath*, an invaluable book by psychiatrists Richard Brown and
Patricia Gerberg, who are also coauthors on many of Dr. Streeter's studies and ex-
perts in the use of breathing as a treatment for mental health disorders such as
PTSD.[23] Participants practiced Coherent Breathing at the end of each yoga session
for twenty minutes at a rate of five breaths per minute.

There were some differences between this dosing study and our earlier research.
For one thing, there was no walking or reading control group to compare with the
yoga practitioners in the dosing study. Additionally, all our participants had been
diagnosed with Major Depressive Disorder and either were not on antidepressant
medication or had been on a stable dose of antidepressant medication for at least
three months before they began their participation. The goal was to discern whether
more yoga practice, measured by more frequent classes and homework sessions, re-
sulted in better emotional health outcomes in a depressed population.

The measurement tool the research team used is called the Beck Depression
Inventory-II (BDI-II), which is a standard assessment tool used by mental health
practitioners.[24] This self-reported questionnaire asks participants twenty-one questions, and it takes less than ten minutes to complete. The higher the score on the
BDI-II, the more severely depressed a person is determined to be.[25]

At the beginning of the twelve weeks, the participants' mean BDI-II scores in-
dicated that they had moderate depression. At the end, when they completed the
BDI-II again, both the low-dose and high-dose groups' scores had lowered by half
or more. A significant number of participants achieved what is called "remission"
of their depressive symptoms, meaning their final BDI-II scores were in the lowest-
scoring category within the test.[26]

Given these results, the study's publication made headlines, like this one in *Time*
magazine: "It's Official: Yoga Helps Depression."[27] It was notable that a significant
number of participants from both the high- and low-dose groups responded so meaningfully. Dr. Streeter concluded that the twice-weekly classes plus home practice

the low-dose group completed may be more accessible to more people because that regimen requires less time and energy but still was shown to offer mood benefits.[28]

The book you are holding in your hands is based on (but is not a full replica of) the sequences of poses and breath work that produced the remarkable results this study achieved. Whatever schedule you are able to consistently and sustainably practice, you can feel confident that the yoga in this book is a meaningful part of your journey toward wholeness.

Study 3: New Horizons in Science, Yoga, and Emotion

At the time of this writing, our team is in the midst of a third study, one that will build on our previous findings to continue to advance our understanding of what impact yoga has on depression and anxiety.

We learned from our first study, with subjects who did not have diagnosed depression or anxiety disorders, that increases in levels of the neurotransmitter GABA were associated with decreased anxiety and improved mood.[29] These benefits were found to be greater for yoga practitioners than for those who completed a walking program that required the same amount of physical exertion as the yoga.

Our second study pressed the question of how much yoga was required to achieve mood-boosting results in people living with clinical depression. The results suggested that individuals with depression who attended yoga classes two to three times per week and did homework reported an improvement in their mood. To reinforce our finding, reviews of what scientists call "randomized controlled studies"—a highly rigorous type of research—that use yoga to treat depression show a range of one to five yoga sessions per week having a positive association with improved mood.[30]

Now, we are setting our sights on the next horizon. Our third study's participants will have Major Depressive Disorder diagnoses, and they will complete the low-dose, twice-weekly yoga program we used in our second study. We will use both self-reported questionnaires and MR spectroscopy to measure changes in both mood and brain chemistry. And we will compare their experiences to a control group of participants who are doing a walking program instead of yoga practice.

As we move through this new research, I don't know what excites me more— the hope that we might discover new and deeper insights into how yoga impacts emotional well-being, or the knowledge that this study's takeaways will urge us on to the next question, the next curiosity, the next step toward understanding the how and why of yoga's impact on the mind. I am inspired by the idea that yoga may hold promise for helping ease the symptoms of your depression or anxiety.

A Deeper Exploration: The Polyvagal Theory

Earlier, we discussed the SNS and the PNS, the two systems that determine whether we are in an active or a resting mode, both physically and mentally. Now, we'll explore a leading edge in scientific research, one that may account for how yoga—breath work in particular—promotes balanced emotions. The idea, which was developed in the 1990s by the preeminent scientist and behavioral neuroscience expert Stephen Porges, is called the polyvagal theory.[31]

The vagus nerve, for which the theory is named, begins at the base of the brain and runs through your thoracic and abdominal cavities. It is part of a circuit that connects to and exerts control over most of your internal organs, conveying electrical impulses to the lungs, heart, abdomen, and digestive tract. The vagus also sends information about the condition of those organs back to your brain.[32] In short, the vagus nerve is a two-way highway that carries most of the information that travels from the body to the brain and back again.

Vagal activity also influences how emotional states express themselves in your physical body.[33] When your vagus nerve is functioning properly, it effectively controls parasympathetic stimulation of your heart, acting as what's called a "vagal brake" that reduces your heart rate and blood pressure and helps you calm down.[34] This effect is believed to be associated with the breath. Scientists who have written about the effects of yoga on the autonomic nervous system theorize that one technique of stimulating the vagus nerve is breathing while contracting your throat muscles, referred to as "resistance breathing," similar to what you will soon learn as "Ocean Breath." Researchers suspect that brief periods of held breath combined with resistance breathing may also increase PNS activity.[35]

So what is "the polyvagal theory," and why is it so exciting for the future of scientific inquiry into yoga and mental health? While scientists previously understood the SNS and PNS to be the entirety of the autonomic nervous system, the polyvagal theory imagines that the PNS is a more complex system in and of itself, elegantly divided into more than one (hence the prefix "poly") component.

The theory proposes that the vagus nerve actually has two major components, one "myelinated" and one not. Myelin is a fatty sheath that covers nerves and makes those nerves conduct impulses faster. Unmyelinated nerves carry impulses more slowly. According

(continues)

(continued)

to Porges, the myelinated circuit is more recently evolved than the unmyelinated one. He argues that the myelinated vagus is a circuit of social interaction—when it is functioning properly, it activates the "vagal brake" in a way that better enables you to remain calm and connected with others, even when faced with a challenge.[36] He also likens the polyvagal theory to a traffic signal—the unmyelinated vagus is the red stoplight indicating an emergency or the yellow warning light putting you on alert, while the myelinated vagus represents the green light of rest, renewal, and social engagement.[37] In other words, it's the myelinated vagus that researchers believe is activated in ways that support positive emotional health. As Porges puts it, "The breath literally turns on and off the myelinated vagus, which supports engagement behavior, positive affective experiences, and relationship building."[38]

In the polyvagal theory, Western science affirms what yoga practitioners have known for millennia—that yoga balances the nervous system and brings us into a state of wholeness and emotional well-being.

DEFINING DEPRESSION AND ANXIETY:
THE WESTERN VIEW

Let's step back and consider what we actually mean when we talk about depression and anxiety. It can be a tricky thing to define a condition of the mind in accurate clinical terms. Just as it would be difficult to describe the color green to someone who can't see it, articulating the experience of depression or anxiety can be tough to get just right.

But of course, accurately understanding our emotions is key to our ability to manage them. Our society has a number of casual terms for emotional challenges—we might say we have the blues, feel stressed out, are spinning our wheels, or are feeling down—but when depression and anxiety become more pervasive companions in our everyday lives, we need more precise language, and it's useful to have guidance from the scientific and medical communities.[39]

We've been talking about research through the lens of brain science, so let's stay there for a moment more. Even for clinicians and researchers, depression and anxiety are highly complex, and scientists' understanding of these conditions is constantly evolving. For a long time, depression and anxiety were believed to be caused by imbalanced brain chemistry—too much or too little of various neurotransmitters triggering the brain to send signals that eventually translate into emotions like sadness, hopelessness, fear, or panic. Scientists are now sharpening this understanding at a rapid pace.[40]

Neurotransmitters like GABA remain highly relevant to the understanding and treatment of depression and anxiety. But a leading edge of brain science research is based on something the neuropsychology community calls "neuroplasticity." This is the concept that through learning or experience, a brain can physically adapt, change, and form new connections. It was only in the late 1990s that researchers first considered that our brains can learn, grow, and change throughout our lifetimes.[41]

The use of yoga as a behavioral—rather than pharmacological—treatment for depression certainly underscores the impact our actions have on our brain health. There is great hope in this notion that positive activities and thoughts can literally change our brains for the better.

Now let's step out of the science lab and into the doctor's office, which you might have visited or might be considering visiting for clarity on your condition. When you do, your doctor will use the medical community's main tool for diagnosing mental health problems—the *Diagnostic and Statistical Manual of Mental Disorders* (DSM). The current edition of the *DSM* contains eight depressive disorders, including Major Depressive Disorder (MDD), which affects more than fourteen million Americans, according to the National Institute of Mental Health.[42] "Anxiety Disorders" covers a family of nine diagnoses. An estimated 31 percent of Americans will experience an anxiety disorder at some point in their lives.[43]

It's important to note that depression and anxiety often go hand in hand; people are often diagnosed with disorders in both categories.[44]

Because Dr. Streeter focused on patients with Major Depressive Disorder in our research, that diagnosis warrants a brief discussion here. To be diagnosed with MDD using *DSM* criteria, a person needs to experience five or more of the following symptoms consistently over at least a two-week period:

1. Depressed mood for most of the day
2. Severely diminished interest in activities that would otherwise be pleasurable
3. Significant weight loss or gain due to changes in appetite
4. Physical agitation or lethargy that is noticeable to others
5. Fatigue or loss of energy
6. Inappropriate feelings of guilt or worthlessness

7. Diminished ability to concentrate or make decisions
8. Recurrent thoughts of suicide, with or without a plan or suicide attempt[45]

I share this with you not to encourage self-diagnosis; in fact, I urge you not to try to diagnose yourself! Depression can manifest in multiple ways, and many people suffer from symptoms but do not meet clinical criteria for a particular diagnosis. But I have listed the MDD criteria here for two reasons. First, I want you to understand the type of depression our study participants were living with. Second, I want to equip you with the information you need to take to the doctor if you feel your depression or anxiety warrants medical care.

The idea of visiting a doctor who consults a manual with the term "mental disorders" in its title can feel intimidating and frightening. But I'm reminded of something the wise Professor Albus Dumbledore told Harry Potter in the now-classic series of novels by J. K. Rowling: "Always use the proper name for things. Fear of a name increases fear of the thing itself."[46]

YOUR JOURNEY TOWARD WHOLENESS

In the yogic view, each person has within themselves a natural state of contentment, peace, and joy. As you will learn in the next chapter, yoga philosophy refers to these things as your "birthright."[47]

In this chapter, you learned quite a bit about the complexity of your brain—and, for that matter, your mind. If this new information is making the idea of accessing that birthright, of finding peace and relief from depression and anxiety, intimidating—that's okay. All I want you to see is that yoga is a profoundly useful tool to help you along your way, no matter if you've been formally diagnosed or if you are just feeling anxious or depressed, from your first tentative steps toward wellness to a wide healing path you can stride along with hope and courage. This path leads to greater energy, deep peace, and the luminous gift of happiness that is within you.

I mentioned earlier in this chapter that my role in Dr. Streeter's research allowed me to explore scientifically what I had always believed intuitively as a yoga practitioner and teacher—that yoga enables, encourages, and supports emotional well-being. The body of research in this area continues to swell with new insights and ideas. So wherever you are here and now, in this present moment, you can rest in the knowledge that this book is grounded not in what I believe might be helpful, but in the yoga sequences our research has shown to result in meaningful positive changes to emotional life.

You have taken a brave and hopeful step by opening this book. Your journey toward becoming whole again has already begun.

CHAPTER 2

HOW YOGA CAN SUPPORT YOUR HEALING JOURNEY

I n this chapter, I'll introduce some yogic general philosophical concepts that can help clarify our goals in practicing yoga for improved mental health—and re-assure you that you have chosen a worthy tool to add to your wellness toolbox. Before we begin, I must note that these philosophical ideas are not researched and documented in the same way as the scientific questions I explored in Chapter 1. Nevertheless, I experience yoga philosophy as a profound source of personal heal-ing, and it informs my approach to the yoga practices in this book.

Fundamentally, yoga philosophy assumes a profound connection between the body and mind, in which the condition of your body reflects your state of mind—and vice versa. When it comes to mental health, body and mind reflect each other in a deeply meaningful way.

Think about your muscles and joints. When you are suffering physically, you can usually identify muscles or joints that are out of alignment or have experienced in-jury. At times like these, they feel tight—holding, clenching, or even buckled in on themselves. In this constricted state, blood, joint fluid, and other energy-delivering physical substances are blocked, with no access to your most hurting places.

Yoga understands the same process to be at work in your emotional life. As Amy Weintraub puts it in *Yoga for Depression*, "Whenever there is depression, there is contraction. Some area of the body or mind is compressed; some area of the emotions is blocked."[1] This is a space issue, an access issue; when the mind has closed around an emotional problem, healing is turned away at the door. The goal of yoga practice, then, is to open ourselves, to provide the space we need to clear obstructions that limit us on our healing journey.

LEARNING TO ACCEPT YOUR JOYFUL BIRTHRIGHT

With confidence that you can begin to clear the blockages that hold you back, let's examine the idea called the "yogic birthright."[2] In the yogic view, each person has within themselves a natural state of contentment, peace, and joy. All anyone needs to do to be entitled to this birthright is to be born! Nothing you can do, think, or feel about yourself can take it away.

But if you are suffering from depression or anxiety, this might feel hard to accept. You might even turn a self-judgmental eye in on yourself, saying, "What's wrong with me that I can't experience peace and happiness?" In times of depression, you might not be able to access your birthright, and you may even doubt that you deserve it.

Remember the yogic notion that emotional challenges are like blockages that, if opened, can become springboards for personal change and growth? I hope this idea can help you release any defeated, self-deprecating thoughts you may be experiencing.

Consider this thought experiment: Imagine you are standing outside your house in a rainstorm, without the key to open your front door. How do you feel? Physically uncomfortable? Wet? Cold? Frustrated? Annoyed with yourself for forgetting your key? You might feel all these things, not to mention feeling resentful at being locked out of the comforts of home, as you peer through a closed window and see an inviting teakettle, cozy blanket, and beckoning sofa.

Within all those thoughts and feelings, though, here's something you would *not* likely feel compelled to say to yourself: "Oh, well, if I can't get into my house, I guess I don't live here anymore." In other words, your home is yours, whether or not you can get into it in this moment. So, too, does your emotional birthright of peace and happiness belong to you, whether or not it feels within reach to you right now.

Of course, it bears mentioning that the key to your house is a cut piece of metal that fits neatly into your door's lock. If you have that one key, you have full access to everything that waits on the other side of the door.

If only emotional wellness were that simple! The truth is, there is no one thing, no "master key" that will free you from the challenges that come with life as an emotional being. But remember—everything you are doing to improve your mental well-being, including reading this book, is part of the healing journey toward clearing the obstructions that hold you back. Each time you take a step toward understanding yourself a bit better—by understanding your brain, mind, and body—you move toward accessing the rich source of peace and contentment that already dwells within you.

The rest of this chapter explores four keys that yoga can provide to help you enter your true emotional home. This home is the place you can return to whenever you need to ease your depression and anxiety. It is the grounded base from which you will engage with your life. These keys help unlock the aspect of your being that is the core of yoga philosophy—your mind. In the next chapter, we turn our attention to your physical body as you prepare for the poses we will practice in the chapters to come.

Key 1: The First Steps on Your Healing Path

In Chapter 1, I introduced you to *The Yoga Sutras of Patañjali*, which is regarded as a sacred text in yoga philosophy. The second chapter of this compilation is called "Practice," and its very first sutra maps out a three-part way to begin to cultivate a focused, balanced, and controlled mind. There are many translations of these three actions, but the ones I like best are:

- Self-discipline[3]
- Self-study[4]
- Surrender[5]

For the purposes of our work together, I understand "self-discipline" to mean having the motivation and determination to be consistent in repeating whatever actions support your healing journey. In yoga, that would start with creating the time for practice, practicing at the same time a few times each week, or committing to a basic sequence of poses and breath work exercises that you practice each time you step onto the mat. Without expectation of perfection or a "one-and-done" result, yoga becomes a consistent source of support that you know you can trust to make a difference in your body and mind.

"Self-study," the second action in Patañjali's list, is fundamental to your journey toward wellness. As I noted in Chapter 1, I do not recommend that you educate yourself about mental health with a goal of diagnosing yourself with a particular condition. On the contrary, the concept of self-study asks you to look inward at your body, your thoughts, your emotions—not with an objective of resolving or diagnosing anything, but with the reassurance that knowledge of your individual patterns, triggers, strengths, and challenges will serve as a springboard to what you need to move toward healing. We will delve more deeply into a particularly helpful aspect of this idea later in this chapter.

The final term in this triad, "surrender," can take on a religious or spiritual connotation if you consider it as Patañjali did—a process of giving yourself over to "the Lord." To me, though, surrender has a broader meaning, regardless of the role spirituality might play in your particular journey. It is a reminder to release, to let go, to stay in the present moment and embrace all aspects of the process of pursuing healing and wellness—the messy parts, the triumphant parts, and all the parts in between. Having a tough day on the mat? Surrender to the idea that tomorrow brings a fresh start. Feeling better than you were this time last week? Surrender to the hope that you'll be able to handle your next setback.

You might even approach the idea of surrender as a scientist would—far from expecting a question to have a single answer, look at each step along your journey as a pathway toward a new set of questions, toward new terrain to explore.

Key 2: Your Mind's Powerful Desire for Harmony

The second key is an idea we will return to again and again throughout the book—it assigns three energetic qualities to everything in the entire universe. According to yoga philosophy, everything, whether it's tangible or intangible, inside you or outside, alive or inanimate, consists of some amount of these three qualities:

- Inertia, heaviness, darkness, and steadiness (*tamas*)
- Passion, desire, effort, and restlessness (*rajas*)
- Balance, peacefulness, and harmony (*sattva*)[6]

These attributes exist in constantly changing proportions in everyone and everything. Although they aren't defined as emotions per se, it's easy to understand how too much *rajasic* energy might contribute to anxiety, in the form of an overactive mind. You can also imagine how too much *tamasic* energy can make you want to crawl in bed for a week under the heaviness and darkness of depression.[7] For our purposes, our goal in yoga practice is to help our minds find the right proportions of activity and inertia, so we can actively participate in our day-to-day lives while also allowing ourselves the downtime required for self-care and self-reflection. Aiming to regulate *tamas* and *rajas* helps us to respond appropriately to different situations and to cultivate our ultimate goal—*sattvic* harmony.

Throughout this book, we will return to this three-pronged idea of energy. All three qualities—*tamas*, *rajas*, and *sattva*—have roles to play in the journey toward emotional wellness.

Key 3: Your Clear, Fearless View of Yourself

The third key takes us more deeply into the philosophical idea of "self-study," which we discussed earlier in this chapter. The ability to accurately identify your thoughts and emotions is a crucial skill. When you use it, you can understand the condition of your mind—whether it needs to calm down so it can rest, or needs to be revved-up so you can fuel your daily activities. Having the skill—and the courage—to look within and understand what your deepest thoughts and emotions have to tell you, without fear, shame, or emotional exhaustion, can be the beginning of self-transformation, an invitation to stand up for yourself and do what you need to bring harmony to your emotions.

Even though yoga philosophy asks us to look directly and honestly at our emotions, I know it can be challenging to do so. Let's give this exercise a try: Sit comfortably, breathe normally, and begin to notice your thoughts and emotions. Don't hold back, just let them come. Welcome them as if they were old friends coming to visit you after many years.[8] Some might not be your favorite guests, but they are all invited into your mind. Offer them seats at an imaginary table, where you can see each of them clearly and take the time to pay attention to them. If you are feeling anxious about looking your feelings in their eyes, remember that you are the host of this gathering—no individual emotion is allowed to take over and run the show.

In Chapter 1, I talked about the fear of naming things. Ask yourself not to be afraid of naming your emotions—in fact, can you feel that in naming a feeling, you might discover an insight you hadn't yet let yourself acknowledge?

Once you've named your challenging emotions, reflect on them a little more deeply, gazing directly into their metaphorical eyes as they sit comfortably at your mental table. Ask yourself these three questions about each emotion, either writing down your answers or just giving yourself a moment to notice whatever thoughts emerge:

- What has the emotion helped you with in your life?
- How does the emotion define you?
- Is the emotion helpful to your life right now?

These processes of self-observation and self-reflection are part of the practice of cultivating "true knowledge," called *viveka* in Sanskrit.[9] This skill allows you to discern what is real, true, and accurate, and what is unreal and unhelpful. Mastering *viveka* can't be done in one sitting, in one hour, or even one week—it takes time. But with patience and practice, you'll realize you can acknowledge your emotions for what they are without fear or judgment.

From there, you will be able to see your emotions clearly and without fear. You'll recognize that your emotions are part of your learned behavior in response to stressful situations, not part of your essential nature. Your essential nature is what Patañjali called "unbounded consciousness," free from the constraints and weight of thoughts and emotions.[10] Sit for a moment and let this idea percolate through your mind. See if you can come to a realization that you are more powerful than your emotions, especially when you take a clear-eyed, fearless look at your thoughts and feelings. You might even feel less uncomfortable welcoming each emotional "guest" to your table.

A Deeper Exploration: Build Your Emotional Vocabulary

Naming your emotions is a skill I encourage you to cultivate, as I first mentioned in Chapter 1. Below, you will find a short emotional vocabulary list you can refer to if you are having a hard time articulating your feelings. This is an incomplete list, to be sure! Feel free to jot down additional emotions you have named in the margins, so you can make this list your own.[11]

COMFORTABLE EMOTIONS	CHALLENGING EMOTIONS
Happiness	Fear
Amusement	Anger
Awe	Anxiety
Contentment	Shame
Gratitude	Contempt
Surprise	Hopelessness
Hope	Envy
Inspiration	Embarrassment
Interest	Guilt
Joy	Hate
Love	Dislike
Trust	Sadness
Pride	Agitation
Serenity	Stress
Confidence	Vulnerability
Peace	Tension
Inspiration	Restlessness
Excitement	Confusion

Key 4: Your Power to Turn Your Emotions Around

Having identified and named your emotions, and having recognized that they do not define you, you can start to change and release those that are not serving you at this moment in your life. But how? This key is the yoga philosophy technique of "cultivating an opposite feeling" as a powerful tool to build better mental health. The Sanskrit name for this teaching is the phrase *pratipaksha bhavanam*, with the first word defined as "opposite side" and the second as "feeling" or "forming in the mind."[12]

Think back on the emotions that came up for you during the exercise we did in the previous section. Choose one that you can identify as challenging, that you do not want to define you, and that you know will not be helpful to your life going forward. It may be an emotion that feels like an obstruction to your happiness, such as anger, discouragement, or jealousy. It's time to explore the emotion further by asking a few more questions:

- What is the "opposite side" of the challenging emotion?
- Does the thought of the opposite emotion bring you a feeling of emotional space and happiness?
- Can you think of concrete ways to start to build this new, opposite feeling to replace the challenging emotion?

We will practice this skill in the chapters to come. When you do, you'll see that by using your self-observant, discerning mind, you have the power to turn a challenging emotion into a constructive, empowering tool for moving forward in your life. Remember what you learned in Chapter 1 about neuroplasticity, the scientific term for how behaviors and thoughts can physiologically change our brains? The Western medical community and the yoga philosophical tradition are aligned around the idea that our mental health is something that we can—through a multifaceted approach—change for the better.

CHAPTER 3

THE LIFE FORCE IN
YOUR BODY

Yoga is an "embodied" practice, meaning it anchors you in your physical body, even when depression or anxiety try to keep your attention stuck in your mind. But in addition to the physical body, the ancient yogis believed in an interactive network of energy patterns we cannot see. We can easily sense them inside our physical bodies, though, when we pay close attention. Think of this chapter as a map of these intricate energetic pathways. I will briefly explore four aspects of your "energetic body" to give you a sense of how complex and elegant the yogic view is. We will return to these concepts throughout the book, reflecting on them as they relate to the emotional attributes we'll explore in each of the practice chapters.

LIFE FORCE—*PRANA*

Yogic philosophy teaches that life force, called *prana*, connects the many aspects of the self. When the layers of our being are open, life force flows easily and fully among them and creates a sense of harmony and balance that can be palpable. But when life force can't flow due to physical, mental, or emotional blockages, energy becomes stagnant, your body becomes fatigued, your emotions may turn dark and brooding, and, well, you just aren't your full self. Once again, you're locked out of your emotional home. When life force flows freely, though, you can build and conserve it, so that you feel fully alive and able to participate in your daily life with a sense of purpose and harmony.

ENERGETIC PATHWAYS—*NADIS*

Life force flows through us via a system of energetic pathways called *nadis*. Depending on which source you read, there are seventy-two thousand or more of these channels.[1] For the purposes of this book, we only need to briefly mention the three widest and most important *nadis*, which envelop the spinal column:

- The "channel of comfort" (*ida*) begins at the base of your spine, on the left.[2]
- The "solar current" (*pingala*) begins at the base of your spine, on the right.[3]
- The "gracious channel" (*sushumna*) travels straight up the spine.[4]

Ida and *pingala* travel up the spine, looping and crossing it—and the *sushumna*—at the first six of your seven energy centers called *chakras*, joining at the "third eye" *chakra* between the eyebrows.[5]

ENERGY CENTERS—*CHAKRAS*

Chakras are psycho-energetic centers, sometimes called "wheels," that dwell within your body at the points along your spine where the major *nadis* cross. Your *chakras* are "whirlpools of energy" that keep your physical body functioning properly by balancing and distributing life force throughout your being.[6] They are not physical points per se, though each occupies its own general region in your body. Like the physical areas in which they reside, *chakras* can be healthy or blocked, fluid or stiff, open or depleted. There are seven major *chakras* located along the central axis of energy in your body—the central *nadi* called *sushumna*. Each *chakra* is associated with a different aspect of your being and is activated by one or more categories of yoga postures and breath. Turn the page for a summary of their effects on your mental and emotional well-being.[7]

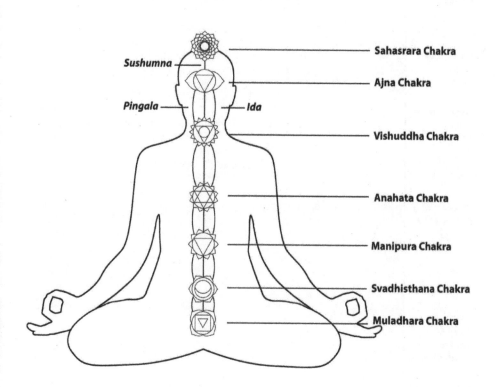

	Sanskrit Name	Location	Emotional Associations	Yoga Poses
Root Chakra (First Chakra)	Muladhara	The base of the spine	Security, safety, and a sense of being connected to the earth	Seated poses and standing poses that cultivate groundedness and stability
Sacral Chakra (Second Chakra)	Svadhisthana	Below the navel, at the sacral area where the spine and hip bones meet	Intimacy, healthy sexuality, desire, and creativity	Forward bends and hip-opening poses
Navel Chakra (Third Chakra)	Manipura	Between the navel and the solar plexus	Self-esteem, personal power, and healthy social interaction	Twists and poses that open and stimulate your abdominal core
Heart Chakra (Fourth Chakra)	Anahata	Behind the heart	Love and healthy expression of emotions. It is your literal energetic "center" because there are three chakras below it and three above it.	Backbends and some standing poses
Throat Chakra (Fifth Chakra)	Vishuddha	Behind the base of the throat	Clarity and purity in verbal communication	Poses that draw the chin and the upper chest toward one another, and poses that create space for your throat, like Supported Reclining Backbend and Standing Backbend
Third Eye Chakra (Sixth Chakra)	Ajna	Behind the intersection of the eyebrows	Insight, inner wisdom, and a calm and focused mental state	Head-down and inverted positions
Crown Chakra (Seventh Chakra)	Sahasrara	The crown of the head	Balance of the mind and a unified consciousness	Inverted positions and meditation

HAND POSITIONS—*MUDRAS*

At moments in the yoga sequences throughout this book, I'll ask you to bring your hands into particular positions called *mudras*. These postures reflect the yogic notion that the positions and movements of your fingers affect the flow of life force within your body. There are many *mudras*, but in this book, I focus most on two that yoga traditions teach to channel life force for physical and mental healing, commonly called Prayer Position and the Gesture of Consciousness.[8]

Prayer Position, or *anjali mudra*, is used as a form of greeting in Indian culture and in some Western yoga classes. In Western yoga practice, the simple yet profound movement of bringing your hands together at the center of your chest is also symbolic of uniting and balancing your body and turning your attention to your heart center. The Gesture of Consciousness, or *chin mudra*, is practiced by bringing the index fingers and thumbs of each hand together to form a circle, then placing your palms on your thighs, facing upward. This *mudra* is symbolic of uniting your mind with your essential, true nature, suggesting that you can contemplate your connection to something larger than yourself, something greater and more profound than your personal story.

HOW YOGA POSTURES CAN CHANGE YOUR MIND

You are getting ready to step onto the mat and begin your yoga practice. For that, you'll need your physical body!

I mentioned in Chapter 1 that only three of Patañjali's 196 yoga sutras involve the practice of physical postures, called *asanas* in Sanskrit. Yet their message is clear and profound—when you practice postures in a steady and comfortable manner, your body can release and relax, and your mind can be drawn into a meditative state.

The physiological changes that occur when you practice yoga postures can help to change your state of mind, so that you come away from extremes of emotions into a place of harmony in your center. As we explore yoga sequences designed to attain specific emotional goals like empowerment or calm, I will return to the philosophical foundation for everything we do in yoga—that our goal in practicing yoga is to relax the body so the mind can come to a place of balance and peace.

As you'll see, yoga postures help release physical restrictions, like tight muscles, and create a sense of spaciousness inside the body. In turn, according to yoga philosophy, life force begins to increase and flow more fully, and your mind has space to grow into, space where it can attend to the physical and energetic sensations within. This begins to align body, breath, and mind, creating a state of embodied connection and integration of your inner and outer bodies. This physical and energetic alignment is fertile ground for transformation.

The yoga posture sequences in our second and third studies were developed by combining different groups of poses for a prescriptive practice to ease symptoms of depression and create a centered mental state. In the next chapter, you'll learn more about how each of these categories of poses can help your healing journey advance. You are now ready to step onto the mat knowing that both Western scientific research and Eastern philosophy support your decision to integrate yoga into your quest for emotional health and happiness.

CHAPTER 4

GETTING READY FOR YOUR YOGA PRACTICE

You have learned a lot about how yoga works from both scientific and philosophical perspectives. Now you are ready to turn your attention to more practical matters that will set you up for a successful experience you can look forward to returning to again and again on your journey toward wellness.

I will start with three practical aspects of your practice—what props to use, when to fit yoga into your day, and how to set up your home practice. From there, we will discuss the structure of each of the five yoga sequences included in this book, explaining the thinking behind why each category of poses was chosen for you.

CHOOSE THE RIGHT YOGA PROPS

You can peruse entire catalogs and websites devoted to yoga props and accessories. But for a successful practice, you really only need a few key items, starting with some comfortable, breathable clothing and bare feet. Having a small set of the right yoga props will give you options for adjustments you can make so that each pose is accessible and comfortable for your body. Here's what you will need:

- **Yoga mat**: This can be made of rubber, vinyl, jute, or even cotton. Choose a mat that feels comfortable on your hands, feet, and body, and that offers enough padding to support your weight without making you feel unstable. Be sure your hands and feet don't slip—your mat should feel slightly sticky.
- **Blocks**: Yoga blocks are typically made of foam, though natural materials like wood or cork are also available. Blocks give you an elevated surface on which to rest your hands in some standing poses, your back in lying-down back-bends, or your head in seated forward bends. There are three positions in which you can place a yoga block—I will refer to them throughout the practice chapters of the book.

     High: Place the block vertically, with its short edge on the floor; in this position it will be about nine to ten inches high.

     Medium: Set the long edge of the block on the floor, so that it is about six inches high.

     Low: Lay the block on the floor on its flat "body," so that it is about four inches high.
- **Belt**: A yoga belt is simply a cloth strap that can be held at its ends by one or two hands in poses that stretch tight legs and hips, or buckled into a loop that can be wrapped around your legs or back for extra support in seated or lying-down poses.
- **Blankets and/or bolster**: For many poses in this book, you will need a few folded blankets to support your body by elevating your hips, cradling your head, or simply covering your body during rest. Your blankets should be firm, unlike the kind of soft blanket you'd use on your bed. You can find blankets commonly used for yoga practice on many yoga accessory websites. If your hips and back like more support, you might also like to have a yoga bolster on hand. A bolster is a long, firm pillow that can cushion your body in a number of ways.

DECIDE WHEN TO PRACTICE

Traditionally, yoga practice is done at transitional times of the day, either morning or evening. This makes sense if you consider how yoga can ease you into your day, awakening your body and mind if you practice first thing in the morning. It also is appealing to think about yoga as a signal to your brain and body that it is time to let go of a long day and shift into a quieter, more restful mode in the evening.

Though the case can be made for both times, challenges also come along with each. In the morning, your mind might be at its most alert, fresh, and clear for the day ahead. But your body might be stiff and sluggish, yearning for a few more minutes under the covers.

By evening time, it can be difficult to find any time for yourself, much less time to practice yoga in a quiet, peaceful space. And although your body is likely more open after a day of moving and doing, your mind may be tired and distracted.

Simply put, the perfect time to practice yoga is the time that feels best to you—the moment in the day when you feel awakened or refreshed, activated or calmed, when your schedule is open enough so your practice doesn't compete with your daily commitments and activities. There will always be challenges that tempt you away from your mat. Your depression might be suppressing your motivation to do much of anything, never mind something physically active or new and different. Or your anxiety might have your mind in such a whirl that you can't imagine being able to calm yourself enough to focus on a meditative practice like yoga.

None of these concerns needs to stop you from moving forward with your practice, though. Instead, you can accept these challenges as part of your healing process. Practicing in the morning might, over time, help your body transition from sleep to wakefulness more smoothly. After a number of evening practices, you might notice sleep comes more easily and that your bedtime thought-swirl slows a bit.

Be reassured—there is a yoga routine you can practice regularly at home. It's simply a matter of looking at what you most need from your practice, looking realistically at your daily schedule, and experimenting with your options for when you can most meaningfully meet yourself on your mat. You should plan for each of the practices in this book to take anywhere from twenty to forty-five minutes, depending on your available time and energy level. Think about how often you can reasonably expect to practice—from one to three times per week is a great initial goal.

SET UP A PRACTICE SPACE

Setting up a home practice space requires very little preparation and maintenance. All you really need is a small space in a quiet room where you can lay out your props, stretch out fully on your mat, and feel calm and grounded enough to fully show up for your yoga. A number of poses in the book ask you to use a wall for support—try to have four to five feet of clear wall space available if possible.

You might like to make your space special by placing a meaningful object like a photograph, a natural element like a pinecone or stone, or anything else that is significant to you somewhere you can see it as you practice. This is not necessary, but it can be a helpful focal point to remind you of your emotional and physical goals in yoga—and in life.

TO CLOSE EYES OR NOT TO CLOSE EYES? LISTEN TO YOUR CUES

There are many times when yoga teachers ask students to close their eyes. This is a deliberate, meditative action meant to turn the sense organs—starting with the eyes—inward, rather than anchoring your senses in the external world. Closing your eyes can bring a well-deserved respite from the distractions of the day, letting you more easily focus on the sensations in your body and your thoughts.

But if you struggle with depression or anxiety, this idea of drawing your attention inside your body and mind might not be a positive experience. With eyes closed, some people can come into a painful state of rumination that often accompanies depression. When they close their eyes, they might immediately think anxiously about everything they didn't get done today, need to do tomorrow, and might have forgotten to add to their to-do list in the first place. Some may suddenly remember a vexing issue at work, at home, or in a relationship, with that inward-facing mind deciding that now, this very moment, is the best and only time to try to solve the problem.

If you can relate to any of these experiences, it may not be productive to close your eyes during your yoga practice. A better option may be to lower your eyelids halfway rather than close them completely. This will help you keep your mind focused because half-open eyes can help keep your mind in the present moment, even as you screen out some external stimuli that could create distractions.

Since moods vary from day to day, "open your eyes" to the state of your mind at the start of each practice, and meet it wherever it is. Practice with your eyes closed or halfway open, whichever creates more focused attention in your mind, so you can cultivate an inner presence that will support your journey into well-being.

YOUR FIVE YOGA PRACTICES

Each of the next five practice chapters offers a short, accessible, and balanced sequence of yoga poses and breath work that is connected to a specific emotional goal: centeredness, empowerment, energy, calm, or balance. As you work through the practices, you will notice that you connect to some when you are struggling with depression and to others when you are feeling anxious.

The sequences are based on the poses that were used in the research I described in Chapter 1, but it's important to note that I have chosen not to replicate the study's sequences exactly. There are a number of reasons for this, including my desire that your practice be accessible to you at home, without a yoga instructor in the room. If you are interested in knowing the full sequence of poses we used in the studies, please refer to the journal article describing the second study for a complete list.[1] In the meantime, the poses in the practice chapters have been selected because I believe they can have a significant positive impact on your emotional health, and they are easily practiced on your own.

Each practice chapter follows a sequence of poses, one from each of the ten categories we used in the studies.

- Centering Pose with Ocean Breath
- Seated or Reclining Pose
- Sun Salutation
- Standing Pose
- Active or Restorative Backbend
- Transition Pose
- Seated Forward Bend
- Inversion
- Deep Relaxation with Ocean Breath
- Coherent Breathing

With the exception of Coherent Breathing, these groups of poses all play an important part in Iyengar yoga as tools to help manage depression and anxiety.[2] In Iyengar philosophy, it is believed that seated poses help to center the mind, Sun Salutation and standing poses move energy and build confidence, and seated forward bends are calming for the mind. Backbends "let in the light," as the Iyengar yoga teacher Patricia Walden puts it, and inversions cultivate emotional stability.[3]

It is important to do a transition pose after a backbend to elongate your spine in a neutral position before you practice a forward bend. And of course, deep relaxation is the wonderful gift you give to yourself after you've made your way through your practice—a well-deserved time of deep rest and restoration for your body and mind.

As you first learned in Chapter 1, Coherent Breathing, a practice that brings inhales and exhales into an even rhythm, helps to balance the stress response of the nervous system.[4] It was practiced at the end of every yoga session during our second study, and it is included in all five practices (Center, Empower, Energize, Calm, and Balance). When you choose one of the sequences in Chapters 5–9, practice the poses that feel most constructive for your emotions. Focus on those that make you feel more grounded, centered, and lighter after your practice. Put aside, for a while, any pose that creates tightness in your body or a heightened sense of dark or brooding emotions, fear, anxiety, or depression. You can practice these poses at other times, when your emotions have shifted and you feel that you will benefit from them.

Now let's delve a little more deeply into the benefits of each pose category.

Centering Pose with Ocean Breath

In your centering pose, you start the journey of moving away from the external world so you can be fully present in your practice. You turn your attention inward and listen for the messages that your body and emotions want, and need, to share with you. You might feel a palpable tightness in your abdomen, your shoulders, or your chest. Taking the time in your centering pose to name and acknowledge the physical sensations in your body will open the door to your inner landscape, and help you to understand what emotions lie within. Ultimately, your practice will lead you from understanding yourself to transforming yourself, at which point new and constructive emotions will replace the judgmental, negative thoughts that hold you back from realizing your potential for a happy, well-balanced life. As you have learned, this process is your parasympathetic nervous system (PNS) doing its calming, stress-managing work.[5]

Each centering pose includes a short practice of Ocean Breath. The ancient yogis practiced yogic breathing, or *pranayama*, because they observed a connection between the quality of the breath and the condition of the mind. In yoga philosophy, Ocean Breath helps open energetic pathways so that life force, or *prana*, is able to move freely through your entire body.

HOW TO PRACTICE OCEAN BREATH

Ocean Breath is a practice you will return to again and again throughout this book, but it's also a practice that is easy to do whenever your nervous system feels jangled and in need of balancing.

You practice Ocean Breath when you slightly contract the muscles of your throat and elongate your breath. It is called Ocean Breath because its sound is reminiscent of an ocean wave softly lapping at a distant shore. Close your eyes for a moment. As you inhale, imagine a wave gently breaking, and as you exhale, visualize the wave softly flowing back into the ocean.

Ocean Breath also sounds like an inner sigh. When practiced correctly, it has an audibly rich, full, resonant vibration that soothes the mind. Ocean Breath is a calming love song that sings directly to your heart. To start your journey into Ocean Breath, you will learn to breathe with an emphasis on elongating your exhalation, which will help quiet your mind and signal your brain to relax. Allow the elongation and vibration of your breath to become your intimate connection to prana, the life force energy that flows through every being.

You'll start Ocean Breath by sitting comfortably on the floor, on a folded blanket, or in a chair—whichever position best allows you to keep your spine tall and chest open. Bring your hands into the Gesture of Consciousness by bringing the tips of your index fingers and thumbs together and resting your hands on your thighs, palms upward. If you are not able to sit comfortably, practice in a reclining position instead, resting your hands on the floor. When you connect your thumb and index finger in the Gesture of Consciousness, you are connecting to your true nature, to the energy that supports and sustains you.

Close your eyes or lower your eyelids, and draw your attention inward. Take a few full, deep breaths, and when you are ready to begin Ocean Breath, follow these steps:

Start with a normal, long inhalation through your nose.
Exhale with your mouth open, creating an audible but soft sighing sound.
Close your mouth and inhale normally.
Exhale through your nose, adjusting how you gently hold your throat muscles so your breath generates a similarly audible, sighing sound.
Let your throat relax, and inhale through your nose.
Continue to inhale normally as you practice the last two steps of Ocean Breath for two to three minutes, emphasizing the gentle "inner sigh" sound of your exhalations.

Once your practice of Ocean Breath exhalations becomes comfortable, see how it feels to practice both inhaling and exhaling in Ocean Breath, creating the soft "inner sigh" sound as you imagine a gentle ocean wave coming onto the shore while you inhale,

(continues)

(continued)

and softly flowing back out to sea as you exhale. If you are challenged by Ocean Breath, please be kind to yourself. Relax with a few normal breaths if your breath feels labored or if you feel tense. Directing your breath in this way does not come easily to everyone, though with continued practice, it will gradually become easier. As the wise meditation teacher and yoga philosopher Sally Kempton is known for saying, the goal in yoga practice is "steady effort in the direction you want to go."[6] Let each attempted Ocean Breath guide you in that direction, as steadily as a tide rolls in each day, without fail.

As you move through the practices in Chapters 5–9, if you feel challenged or overwhelmed by Ocean Breath, or if you find that your mind begins to ruminate on difficult emotions, simply move on to focus on practicing the postures. With practice, you will become comfortable and proficient, able to practice Ocean Breath with ease. When you are finished, sit quietly and observe the quality of your mind and emotions.

Seated or Reclining Poses

Your seated or reclining pose will awaken and warm up your body in preparation for your practice. When you sit in a comfortable posture with your spine tall, your physical body is stable and grounded, while your chest lifts and opens. You will feel yourself supported by the earth, and at the same time you will feel a sense of lightness in your torso, allowing breath to flow freely throughout your body, especially nourishing your lungs and heart, the vital organs associated with the flow of energy through your body.

Some of the seated poses include raising your arms overhead. Patricia Walden often relates a story about how her teacher, the yoga master B. K. S. Iyengar, instructed his students who were suffering from depression: "If you keep your armpits open, you'll never get depressed."[7] Since Iyengar was not a physician, his suggestion was not backed by medical evidence. Taking his suggestion at face value, it may sound, well, simplistic, especially to anyone in a state of deep suffering. But through yoga practice, he understood what the ancient yogis believed—that by opening the energetic pathways in the body, the heart and lungs, essential to our physical and emotional well-being, are opened and brought into a state of optimal functioning. When you practice poses that involve opening or raising your arms throughout the practice chapters ahead, perhaps you'll feel more air coming into your lungs, more breath flowing through your body, or more spaciousness around your heart. Perhaps these feelings will help you to feel more alive and balanced, relieved of some of your suffering.

Sun Salutation

Sun Salutation is a "flow," a set of movements meant to further warm up and energize your body and breath. You will practice Sun Salutation in each practice chapter, setting an intention that aligns with the emotional goal of that chapter. It is one of the most common physical practices in many yoga styles, including Iyengar yoga.

While there are many variations of Sun Salutation, the intention of each style is similar—to connect yourself to the rhythm of the natural world as you honor the life-giving presence and power of the sun. When you practice Sun Salutation, you connect yourself to nature; you become part of the continuum of the universe.

When your mind is in an overactive state and you find it hard to settle your body and mind down, Sun Salutation "meets the energy of the mind," in Patricia Walden's phrasing.[8] When you're feeling lethargic and taking action is difficult, Sun Salutation can help build up and restore your energy, so you can actively participate in your daily life. Over the next five pages, you will learn how to practice Sun Salutation. Once you are comfortable with the instructions, you can turn to pages 172–173 for a two-page refresher to cue you through the flow.

How to Practice Sun Salutation

Here is our Sun Salutation sequence. I've included a few pointers for each pose to help you align your body and move with your breath from one pose to the next. If you are a beginner, I suggest practicing each pose separately once or twice before you combine them into a flow.

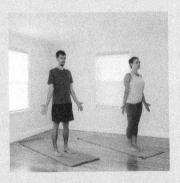

Mountain Pose

Ground your feet fully into the earth. Feeling the stability and firmness of your feet, lift up through your whole body, with your ankles, knees, hips, shoulders, and ears aligned one over the other. Feel your legs, hips, and torso awakening with energy. Imagine a helping hand just above your head, helping you to lift upward from the base of your spine through the crown of your head.

Take one breath, noticing how your physical body lifts upward from earth into your heart as you inhale, and draw your attention from the crown of your head down into your heart as you exhale.

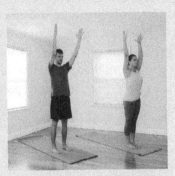

Upward Hand Pose

As you inhale again, reach your arms upward. Stretch completely through your arms, hands, and fingers, and feel your arms awakening with the flow of prana. Bring your arms as much in line with your ears as possible, to elongate and open your chest (and your armpits!).

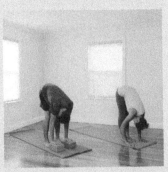

Standing Forward Bend Pose

As you exhale, fold forward from your hip joints and bring your hands to your shins or the floor, or rest them on blocks. As your trunk draws downward, notice that your mind draws inward. Standing forward bends can calm an anxious or scattered mind.

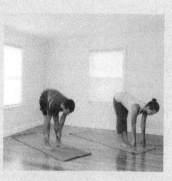

Standing Forward Bend Pose—Head Up

Inhaling, lift your trunk up until your back is flat, placing your hands on your shins or on the floor. Stretch your trunk forward. Look forward, or gaze at the floor for more relaxation in your neck.

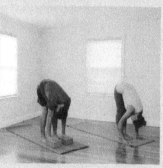

Standing Forward Bend Pose

Exhaling, lower your trunk toward the earth once more, grounding your hands on your shins or the floor or resting them on blocks.

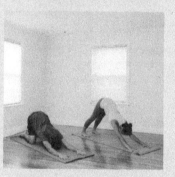

Downward Facing Dog Pose

As you inhale, bend your knees and place your hands on the floor. As you exhale, step your feet back and stretch through your arms, shoulders, and spine. Lift your hips up toward the ceiling so your body forms a triangle with your hips at the apex, coming into Downward Facing Dog Pose, or place your knees on the floor in a modified position, for less stress in your wrists or shoulders. Remain in the pose for three breaths.

With each inhalation, reach upward through your wrists, arms, and trunk, all the way to your hips, and enjoy a sense of spaciousness through your upper body (and, again, your armpits!). As you exhale, let your hips draw away from your head and feel any tension in your shoulders releasing. With each exhalation, reach downward through your legs, pressing your heels toward earth. Don't worry whether your heels actually touch the floor; it's the action of reaching through your legs that awakens them and creates stability throughout your body.

(continues)

(continued)

High Plank Pose

From Downward Facing Dog Pose, inhale and bring your shoulders over your wrists, letting your hips descend slightly to come into line between your legs and your trunk. For more support, place your knees on the floor.

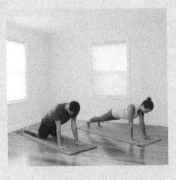

Four Limb Staff Pose

As you exhale, bend your elbows back toward your feet and lower your body toward the floor, with your knees either on or off the floor. Then lower your body all the way to the ground, coming onto the tops of your feet.

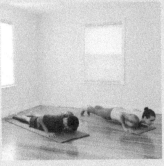

Cobra Pose or Upward Facing Dog Pose

While inhaling, slowly lift your trunk upward and open your chest, staying grounded through your feet, legs, and hands as you come into Cobra Pose. You can stay in Cobra and enjoy a feeling of opening and lifting your heart, or, if your back is comfortable, you can lift your hips and legs off the floor as well, coming into Upward Facing Dog Pose, keeping your hands and feet in contact with the ground. Let your heart lift and notice the openness across your chest.

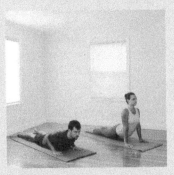

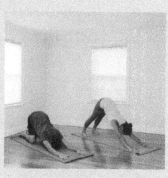

Downward Facing Dog Pose

While exhaling, turn your toes under, lift your hips up and back, and return to Downward Facing Dog Pose for three breaths.

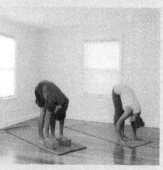

Standing Forward Bend Pose

As you inhale, step your feet forward between your hands. Place your hands on your shins, on the floor, or on blocks and exhale, letting your trunk release down toward the earth.

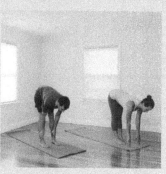

Standing Forward Bend Pose—Head Up

Lift your trunk upward while inhaling, and place your hands on your shins or the floor.

(continues)

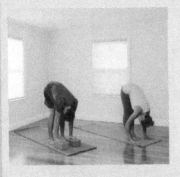

Standing Forward Bend Pose

While exhaling, lower your trunk once again toward the earth, finding a place of quiet in your heart. Place your hands either on your shins, on the floor, or on blocks.

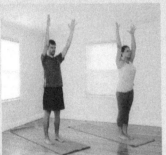

Upward Hand Pose

As you inhale, and with firmness in your legs, raise your torso and your arms upward. If you have a sensitive lower back, bend your knees slightly and place your hands on your thighs as you make this transition.

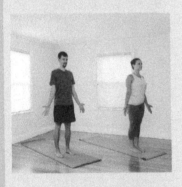

Mountain Pose

As you exhale, bring your arms down by your sides. If you'd like, bring your palms together at your heart center in Prayer Position, a hand gesture that symbolically balances the energies of the right and left sides of your body.[9]

Now you've completed one round of Sun Salutation. Stand in Mountain Pose quietly and notice the effects of your practice. Perhaps your body feels energized, your breath feels freer and more balanced, and your mind has quieted down. Repeat Sun Salutation for one more round, noticing that as each pose becomes more familiar, your body needs less instruction from your mind, and you can stay more focused on the flow of breath and life force throughout your being.

Standing Poses

Standing poses strengthen your legs, open your hips, lengthen your spine, and broaden your chest. In these poses, you build physical stability, your body starts to awaken, and life force begins to flow. You'll soon feel how the poses ignite your body and move stagnant energy, which is especially helpful during times when you feel frozen or unable to take an action, or when your mind can't stop ruminating. You will find openness in your chest and your breath will strengthen. The energy and confidence you build in your standing pose practice follows you off the mat into your life.

Backbends

Backbends have been shown to be helpful for depression and anxiety.[10] They open and release tension in the chest, diaphragm, and abdomen, breaking open the energetic "body armor" that tends to form around the chest in depression and anxiety. You'll cultivate self-empowerment, and you'll notice and learn to express the deepest feelings in your heart in a loving and compassionate way as you release tension in your chest.

There are two different types of backbends in the practice chapters. One is restorative backbends—in Chapters 5, 6, 8, and 9—in which your body is supported by props, allowing you to simply relax into the pose. Restorative backbends open your chest and heart and help to release tension in your diaphragm and abdomen. They are used in the Iyengar yoga tradition to help both depression and anxiety by promoting slow, deep, and even breathing.[11]

You'll practice more active backbends in Chapters 7 and 8. In addition to opening and releasing tension in the front of your body, active backbends tone and strengthen your spinal muscles, core, hips, and legs. Imagine your strong spine staying tall as you move through your day with a feeling of dignity, and the empowerment that comes with the ability to breathe easily and evenly all day long. These advantages can become more accessible when you regularly practice backbends.

Transition Poses

I always recall the maxim "Every action has an equal, opposite reaction" when I think about transition poses. When you do active work in yoga, it's important to undo any tension that might have come into your body by practicing an opposite movement. But if you snap directly from a backbend into a forward bend, you leave yourself vulnerable to discomfort and even injury without a transition pose to ease your body from one position to the next.

After you practice backbends, your transition poses will elongate and release your spine before you move into your seated forward bends. Throughout the practice chapters, you'll practice gentle twists or side stretches to lengthen your muscles and release tension. These transition poses are simple movements, deliberately placed in the sequence to recalibrate your body and ease you into the poses that follow.

Transitions are sometimes difficult in life, especially when you feel challenged to put one foot in front of the other. As you practice these poses, notice what it feels like to smoothly shift from one to the next. Let yourself enjoy that sense of gentle change, and ask yourself how you might cultivate a similar feeling when your life asks you to be resilient and adjust to new realities. Keeping your mind focused on the sensations within, seek out the inner intelligence that will guide you in each pose and in your life. This wisdom will become the bridge that takes you from depression or anxiety into wellness.

Seated Forward Bends

Moving into a forward bend toward the end of your practice is meant to be calming and soothing. Forward bends stretch and release tension all along the back body, in your legs, hips, spine, shoulders, and neck. Many people find seated forward bends calming for anxious, scattered, or ruminating minds, as the poses support you in letting go of distractions. Forward bends offer an opportunity for you to turn your eyes, ears, and mind within so that you can try to see, hear, and understand yourself more clearly.

Like closing our eyes in yoga (discussed earlier in this chapter), forward bends can be emotionally challenging for some. As soothing and calming as forward bends can be, they can also produce some contrary feelings, especially if your mind is overactive and you can't imagine how you will be calm enough to even approach the pose. If you avoid practicing forward bends because uncomfortable emotions surface, I suggest trying a few modifications that can make them more enjoyable, perhaps enough so that you'll look "forward" to your next forward bend practice.

To begin, I recommend you experiment with whether or not to support your head. I've suggested a mixture of options in the practice chapters, so you can discover what is most comfortable for you. Supporting your head can be extra calming and soothing, unless it's difficult for you to close your eyes fully, look downward, or come completely away from the external world. Ultimately, your decision to support your head or close your eyes—or do neither—is completely within your power. Honor your emotions, and let them tell you what is most helpful. A few other modifications that can help you to enjoy forward bends are:

• If the muscles in your hips or the backs of your thighs feel tight, or if your lower back aches after forward bends, start with your knees bent so your trunk hinges at your hip joints, rather than curving over from your mid-spine.
• If it's difficult for you to hold your feet or shins, wrap a belt around your feet and hold the ends of the belt.
• Place your legs a little apart from each other to accommodate the shape of your abdomen and trunk.

Inversions

Inversions—being either upside down or positioned such that your heart is elevated above your head—aid in bringing the body into a state of relaxation, which helps balance the nervous system.[12] The main inversion in each practice chapter is called Inverted Pose. It is accessible to practitioners of any and all skill levels, and I will offer ways it can be modified to suit particular individual needs. Inverted Pose releases tension in the chest, diaphragm, and abdomen. It gently stretches the muscles of your legs, hips, and spine. Your nervous system comes into a resting state by virtue of the fact that you are lying down. Perhaps you'll also notice that when you practice Inverted Pose, your exhalations become slower and longer than your inhalations. In yoga philosophy, Inverted Pose is considered to be a calming pose for the nervous system.[13]

Since posture can affect our emotions, going into an inversion can be an agent for mental change. I say that from personal experience; whenever I need to change my mood, I put myself into an inversion. Remaining quietly in the pose for a few minutes, I feel a palpable shift in my emotions—at the very least, my mind quiets down. Many times, though, I am able to benefit even more, discovering a different way of looking at a relationship or situation in my life, or finding new ways I can be more constructive, helpful, and compassionate toward both others and myself.

Deep Relaxation with Ocean Breath

The last pose in each practice is Deep Relaxation, and as its name suggests, its goal is to completely rest and replenish your physical body and soothe your nervous system. Deep Relaxation is vitally important to give your body time to assimilate and integrate the physiological changes you have created during your practice. This isn't just a New Age claim; scientific studies are discovering that relaxation practices induce changes to our bodies right down to the cellular level.[14] As I noted in Chapter 1, the relaxation response helps to alleviate symptoms of depression and anxiety. It also positively affects factors such as heart rate, blood pressure, oxygen consumption, and brain activity.[15] Taking the time to relax at the end of your practice imprints these physiological changes on your body, thus helping you to feel better from yoga practice for some time after you step off the mat.

Deep Relaxation is your special time to be with yourself. As preparation for your practice, acknowledge your present state of mind and recognize that you have taken time and effort to care for your body, your mind, and your emotions. You have honored your own existence. You are on the path that leads out of the darkness and into the light.

In each practice chapter, you will place a bolster or folded blankets under your knees to help your legs relax, and you will support your head on a folded blanket to help relax your neck. Here are some additional tips for a comfortable Deep Relaxation practice:

- If your lower back enjoys a gentle backbend, place a folded blanket lengthwise under your spine to lift and open your chest.
- If you are comfortable with closing your eyes, use an eye pillow to place very gentle pressure on your eyes and help them relax.
- Close your eyes halfway if closing them completely brings you to a fearful or anxious state of mind.
- If your fingers and toes cannot stop moving, cover them with a blanket or small towels to encourage them to let go.
- Cover your whole body with a blanket to stay warm.

Don't hesitate to change your position if your body is uncomfortable; because your Coherent Breathing practice directly follows Deep Relaxation in each practice chapter, you'll be lying down for another five to fifteen minutes.

Coherent Breathing

Breathing with elongated inhalations and exhalations is part of many traditional yoga methods of breath practice, or *pranayama*. While Ocean Breath is a form of "resistance breathing," in which the throat muscles are slightly contracted to elongate the breath (the inhale, the exhale, or both), Coherent Breathing is defined by the evenness of each breath in and breath out, and it does not include a contraction of the throat muscles.

This practice, which is not from the classical yoga tradition, has been studied by independent researcher Stephen Elliott, who found a correlation between bringing the breath into an even rhythm, and increased blood flow and nervous system balance. He called it "Coherent Breathing" because as the breath approaches an optimally slow rate and depth, it brings the stress-response system into ideal balance.[16]

In our study, participants practiced twenty minutes of Coherent Breathing at a rate of five breaths per minute, at the end of each session, right after their practice of Deep Relaxation with Ocean Breath. Some participants eagerly lay down and easily got through the entire twenty minutes. Other participants had a much more difficult time.

Vincent, a student at a highly competitive university, had such an experience. The first time I supervised him during Coherent Breathing, he seemed to enjoy it well enough to get through the whole practice. The second time, though, it was difficult for him to lie still; at one point, he opened his eyes and told me he just had to move. We took a break, he stretched his arms and legs and shook the tension out of his body. It helped—he made it through the rest of the twenty-minute practice. At the next session, he said he realized that sometimes he was just too anxious to lie still for that long, and that since his mood varied so much from day to day, so did his body's ability to lie still. He could slow his breath to five breaths per minute without issue, but his body was still finding a way to express the variable state of his emotions.

One objective in Coherent Breathing is for our minds to be engaged—present to the flow of each breath. Vincent's mind was distracted by his body, so he was unable to focus on his breath. We experimented with a ten-minute practice that was successful. Building on his confidence that his body could be still for the ten minutes, we gradually increased his Coherent Breathing time until, just two weeks later, he was able to complete the full twenty minutes of Coherent Breathing without a problem. Having become aware of how his body was expressing his emotional state, he had learned to keep his mind focused on his breath so his anxious thoughts—and his body—could quiet down.

Like Vincent, you should make it a habit to acknowledge the state of your emotions, which vary from day to day, before you begin your practice. Just as your emotional state is always in motion, the length of your practice should be similarly flexible.

Empower yourself to set a time limit and breath rate that works for your body and mood. You can start with five to ten minutes of Coherent Breathing, and over time, work your way up to fifteen or twenty minutes. You can always step back to a shorter practice when your mind can't stay focused and present. You should also note that depending on your height, the optimal length of your breath rate will vary between three and one-half breaths and six breaths per minute. A tall person will have a slower optimal breath rate than a smaller or average-height person.[17]

Most people can start by experimenting with five breaths per minute, which is a six-second inhale and a six-second exhale. You can get a CD, download an mp3 file, or download an app to help track this breath rate. The website Coherence (https://coherence.com) offers a number of resources that can guide you. Alternatively, you can set a timer on your phone or stopwatch for the intervals that you are attempting. Remember to keep an open, experimental attitude as you seek the ideal rate for you.

The most important outcome of a Coherent Breathing practice is the realization that your breath has the power to change and regulate your emotions. Once you feel this in your body, you'll be eager to practice it, and it will become a reliable ally on your journey into mental and emotional balance.

Now that you are inspired (we hope!) to bring your yoga practice to life on your very own mat, let's get started with the first practice, in which you will journey toward your emotional center.

YOGA PRACTICES FOR
DEPRESSION AND ANXIETY

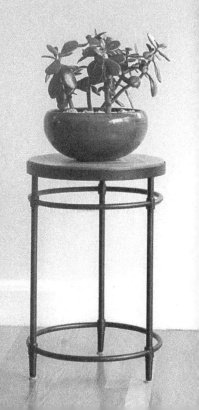

CHAPTER 5

CENTER

A focused mind leads to your true center.

S it quietly, closing your eyes if you feel comfortable doing so, or lowering your eyelids halfway, and bring your palms together in front of your heart.

This movement, which may feel familiar to you or be outside your comfort zone, is called Prayer Position. As I discussed in Chapter 3, Prayer Position is a traditional Indian cultural greeting that honors the sacred spirit within each person. It is often used with the same meaning in Western yoga practice. In some Western yoga classes, placing your hands in Prayer Position is also a way to symbolically set an intention of bringing yourself into a state of connection, where your mind is focused inward and stays present to arising sensations and emotions. In my classes, I often accompany Prayer Position with the direction, "Now come to your center."

These sound like simple words, but they can really challenge some people. Spending time in your center means being secure in yourself—your mind, your body, your entire being. In Prayer Position, your hands press together at your midline, resting against your heart center. But when I give the deceptively straightforward instruction to "come to your center," some people's brains become overactive, turning to the uncomfortable thought, "What if I can't find my center?"

In class, Lillian struggled with this. She would sit down on her blanket and immediately start to fidget. She would change the cross of her legs a number of times, fuss with her hair, adjust her clothes, sigh, and scratch her head. Her anxiety simply wouldn't let her sit still long enough to connect with the emotional and physical center she was seeking. But just a few weeks into her practice, I noticed a distinct change in Lillian's body language. Now she crossed and uncrossed her legs just once, after which they became still. She turned her head from side to side, and then gently tilted her head toward her heart. Her hands remained steady in Prayer Position. When she opened her eyes at the end of the centering meditation, I noticed that her face seemed more relaxed, and her gaze was steadier. One day, she smiled broadly and said, "I just realized there is a place of calmness inside of me." The simple practice of sitting and working with the intention of becoming centered was the beginning of profound changes for her. Like Lillian, you can also cultivate the ability to be still long enough to connect with a meaningful center point within yourself. But as you will soon discover, your "center" is really more than one thing. There's nothing simple about coming to your center, but it is a deeply worthwhile experience to journey toward it.

WHAT IS YOUR CENTER?

The Merriam-Webster Dictionary offers two definitions of "center": (1) the middle point or part of something, and (2) a source from which something originates.[1] In yoga traditions, one's center, or perhaps I should say "centers," fit these definitions perfectly. As the first definition suggests, the midline of the body is the center of the physical self, from the point on the floor that's midway between your feet, to the center of your pelvic floor, up through your trunk to the center of the crown of your head.

The second definition—"center" as a source from which something originates—is also found in yoga philosophy. As I described in Chapter 3, each person's body has a central energy channel along the spine, which is considered to be the main source from which *prana*, or life force, moves throughout our being. Along this channel, each of us also has energy centers called *chakras*. Each *chakra* is a place where energy gathers and then moves through our bodies. And so, as you can see, in the yogic view, we have many centers. Exploring them is one of the most interesting and fruitful aspects of practicing yoga, and it is a key component of how yoga offers tools for healing depression and anxiety.

HOW CENTERING HELPS EASE DEPRESSION AND ANXIETY

Centering the mind leads you first into your thoughts and emotions. I like to say that a centered mind is where you meet yourself. Its value for helping depression and anxiety is that it makes you aware of the content and quality of your thoughts and of the habitual ways your mind operates. You may realize that some of your thoughts have a particularly strong hold on you, and from there you may realize that some emotions are helpful to you, while others can be hurtful and self-defeating. As you learn to respond to thoughts and emotions with equanimity, your emotions gradually lose their hold over you. From a centered, grounded place, you are focused enough to explore your feelings without being overwhelmed by them.

"Easier said than done," you might be thinking. And you're right—when your thoughts are racing or you are feeling the weight of depression in your heart, you may feel that your center is a place you might never reach. Give yourself permission to feel that way—and try to let that feeling go by, remembering that becoming centered is a step-by-step journey rather than an all-or-nothing proposition.

The first step on your journey into centeredness is to be self-observant. When I said before that centering is where you meet yourself, I meant it—your whole self, including thoughts and feelings you might wish you didn't have. Your goal in centering is to listen—to your thoughts, your mood, and your emotions. As hard as they may be to live with, all emotions—especially the challenging ones—are valid and valuable, catalysts for action that can lead to self-empowerment.

The Buddhist meditation teacher Thich Nhat Hanh offers a beautiful image of how to change our relationship to challenging emotions: "You calm your feeling just by being with it, like a mother tenderly holding her crying baby."[2] As parents know and anyone can imagine, a baby is pure feeling, uninhibited from expressing herself in a way that will get her needs met. When we experience a baby's expressions of emotions, we are compelled to feel interested and curious, wanting to understand the source of the emotions and respond in a helpful way.

In centering, we approach our adult emotions with that same openness and curiosity. When I ask you to find your center by closing your eyes and bringing your attention into your body, I am asking you to observe inner sensations and feelings. Draw your awareness away from the external world and visualize the midline of your body, inhaling through that midline down to your feet, and exhaling from your feet through the crown of your head. Identifying your center is the beginning of the journey into connection of mind, body, and breath.

WHY YOUR TRUE CENTER IS A PLACE OF PEACE

Important as this beginning is, it is just that—a starting place from which to launch a deeper journey. Our next step is to find something profound inside yourself—a deep and ultimate peace that is always present in the heart of all beings. The more you practice yoga, the more you develop an internal awareness that connects with your abiding peace. Remember, your center is both a place in your body and a source of profound energy and serenity.

Once you connect with your peaceful center, you can draw upon it at any time, whether you're practicing yoga or cooking dinner; whether you are wondering how you will get through another day with an anxious, overactive mind or feeling painfully disconnected under the weight of depression.

Keep this idea of deep inner peace in mind as you move through the yoga sequence in this chapter, remembering that the whole purpose of practicing yoga is to consciously let go of physical and mental tension and connect with a universal and abiding serenity. With consistent practice, that peace will begin to emerge through the layers of your body—from your center. You will start to trust that this deep peace is available to you as a reservoir of nurturing and calming energy that you can use to help regulate your moods.

An overactive mind, an agitated or distracted mind, or a downward-spiraling mind can all be transformed into a centered, peaceful mind by practicing singular focus, something yogis call "one-pointedness."[3] In this quiet, focused state, your center gives you the ability to hold your mind steady instead of feeling pushed and pulled or overwhelmed by emotions. In this chapter, you'll practice poses that cultivate a focused mind and a grounded body, the two "centers" we have discussed so far. Keep in mind that the two are intrinsically connected—a centered mind cannot be accessed without a grounded body, and the ability to ground your body asks your mind to become focused and centered.

THREE QUESTIONS TO PREPARE YOU FOR PRACTICE

Before you practice this sequence, spend a moment reflecting on these three questions. Observe your feelings in a mindful and curious way. Without judgment, accept and acknowledge your feelings as you move through your practice.

1. Where is your center? Do you feel connected to it, distant from it, or in search of it?
2. Imagine "meeting yourself" at your center. How would you describe yourself?
3. What one word, feeling, or image would you like to focus on during your practice?

Turn the page to start your centering practice. After you practice, you'll check in with yourself again and observe any differences in your thoughts and feelings. Perhaps your whirring thoughts will be quieter and calmer. Perhaps your dark thoughts will be a little lighter, and perhaps the deep inner peace that lives in your center can illuminate the beauty of your heart.

YOGA PRACTICE FOR CENTERING

1. Cross-Legged Seated Pose with Ocean Breath

Sit comfortably with your legs crossed on the floor or on a folded blanket, or sit in a chair if it calls to you. Your spine should be long, and your chest should be broad and open. Place your fingertips beside you and press gently into the floor or the chair to lift your trunk upright; then bring your hands into Prayer Position. Take a moment to visualize the centerline of your trunk, like a soft ray of light rising up from the base of your hips all the way to the crown of your head. Imagine this centerline as a source from which energy emanates throughout your body, equally to the front and back, from side to side, down through your base, and up to the crown of your head.

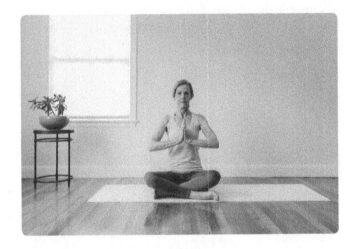

Take a few moments to notice the quality of energy in your body, breath, and mind. Are your limbs quiet and relaxed, or do they keep wanting to move around, fidgeting and futzing like Lillian did during her first few weeks of practice? Do you feel, in other words, "off-center?" In your seated position, encourage your limbs to become quiet. Feel your legs grounding, your arms becoming passive. Breath by breath, feel your arms and legs beginning to rest.

Now notice your breath. Can you visualize a clear, well-defined path for your breath, or is it swirling around inside your body without direction? Visualizing an inner center point inside yourself, breathe into it and breathe out from it. Notice how much calmer your breath becomes once it has a clear path to your center. Finally, notice your thoughts. Are they focused inward, or are they pulled outward by the seemingly endless distractions of your day? Ask your mind to follow your breath into and out of your center, and notice that as time goes by, your mind becomes more interested in finding the still point within your center than in following outward trails of thought.

Now that you've begun to center yourself, you'll practice Ocean Breath to deepen your experience even further.

Ocean Breath can help calm your emotions and center your mind. Take a long, normal inhale. Gently contract your throat muscles to create the sound of an "inner sigh" with your exhale. By elongating your exhalations, you will increase your ability to move away from emotional extremes and to come into your center, where you can exist "undisturbed by dualities."[4] When you are grounded in your center, you may become less swayed by the push and pull of depression and anxiety.

You will remember that Ocean Breath helps regulate the stimulation of your central nervous system—the sympathetic nervous system (SNS), which is action-oriented and responsible for the fight-or-flight response, and the parasympathetic nervous system (PNS), which is calming and restorative, the body's tool for its social engagement and rest-and-digest functions. For a review of how to practice Ocean Breath, see page 39.

Join your index fingers and thumbs together and rest your hands, palms facing upward, on your thighs in the Gesture of Consciousness. Close your eyes or lower your eyelids, and imagine a pendulum swaying evenly from side to side. As it does, visualize how it briefly pauses as it passes through the center point between its two extremes of movement. This is called the position of equilibrium, the perfect center between two equal sides.

Now, observing your breath, visualize that each time you inhale, an "inner pendulum" swings to one side, and as you exhale in an extended Ocean Breath, it swings to the other side, a little more slowly and for longer than it does when you inhale. Visualize the pendulum pausing for a moment at the point between each inhale and exhale. Practice for two to three minutes and then return to normal breathing. Take a few moments to observe the sensations in your body and the feelings in your mind, and feel how you can quickly direct your mind toward a centered state by elongating your exhalations in Ocean Breath. Once you are comfortable practicing Ocean Breath exhalations, practice this exercise with both Ocean Breath inhalations and exhalations.

2. Seated Upward Hand Pose

Remain in Cross-Legged Seated Pose or in your chair and, inhaling deeply, stretch your arms straight up over your head, coming into Upward Hand Pose. Reach upward from the sides of your waist all the way up to your fingertips. Bring your arms down to your sides as you exhale, and notice a quiet pause in your body at the end of the movement. Repeat Upward Hand Pose two more times. Each time, notice how the energy of your physical body increases as you lift your arms upward, and how your

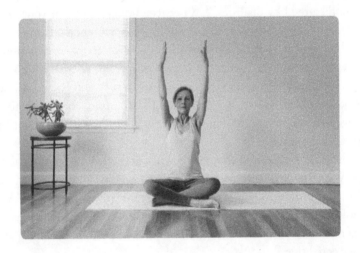

mind quiets down as you exhale. Feel the uplift of your physical body and notice how that lifting sensation affects your emotions. After you finish practicing Upward Hand Pose, bring your hands into Prayer Position and honor that return to your center, where upward and downward energies meet; where body, breath, and mind unite; and where the push and pull of depression and anxiety come to a still point.

3. Centering Sun Salutation

Begin by standing tall in Mountain Pose. Just as you did in Cross-Legged Seated Pose, visualize the centerline of your body, this time from your feet up to the crown of your head. Now let your mind be drawn to the fourth *chakra* (*Anahata chakra*), the area behind your heart, where your emotions reside. As you move through Sun Salutation, breathe into your heart *chakra*, imagining it receiving your inhalation, and then breathe out from it, allowing your exhalation to reach all the parts of your body. Notice how your mind responds when your body is connected to your center of energy—do your thoughts become softer and perhaps easier to process? Practice Sun Salutation while keeping your focus fixed on this center of energy, feeling the movement of your body and your breath in, around, and through it. Experience your body starting to flow through the poses with a sense of integration, with all the parts of your body, the flow of your breath, and your mind connected and centered.

See pages 172–173 for a photographic Sun Salutation refresher.

Mountain Pose
Upward Hand Pose
Standing Forward Bend Pose
Standing Forward Bend Pose—Head Up
Standing Forward Bend Pose
Downward Facing Dog Pose
High Plank Pose
Four Limb Staff Pose
Cobra Pose or Upward Facing Dog Pose
Downward Facing Dog Pose
Standing Forward Bend Pose
Standing Forward Bend Pose—Head Up
Standing Forward Bend Pose
Upward Hand Pose
Mountain Pose

4. Tree Pose

Tree Pose is a standing pose that asks for physical stability as you become grounded into the earth through one foot and stand on one leg. You will need a centered and focused mental state to support your body while it finds steadiness.

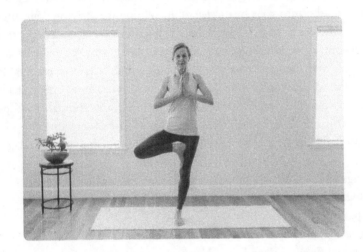

Prepare for Tree Pose by standing with your feet a few inches apart, pressing your feet evenly into the floor, and feeling the stability of the earth beneath your feet. While inhaling, lift up from the center of your arches through the center of your legs and trunk, all the way up to the crown of your head. Let that feeling of stability rise beyond your body, into your heart and mind. You should feel very secure and very aware of your physical center. If you feel unsteady, start with your feet farther apart, or stand with your back against a wall and use it for support.

Now it's time to transform into a beautiful, growing tree. Bend your right knee and come onto the toes of your right foot. Then place your right foot anywhere along your inner left leg. Don't worry about drawing your foot all the way up to your thigh; simply find a point—anywhere except against your knee—where your foot can stay on your left leg without struggle, so you'll be able to enjoy standing steadily on one foot. Bring your hands to heart center in Prayer Position, and focus your attention on this center. Gaze at a point in front of you to help you maintain balance.

Inhale and reach your arms up toward the sky while staying grounded to the earth through your left foot. Feel your heart center being nourished by the sunlight that's filtering through your "branches," and visualize a flower in your heart opening, cupping the luminous energy of your heart.

Hold your pose for ten to fifteen seconds, and then slowly bring your hands down into Prayer Position. Place your right foot on the floor. Repeat the pose, this time lifting your left foot off the floor.

Can you feel more awareness of your center, and of the energy within it? It is a place of stability that allows you to be in the world without being pulled and pushed by it; a place from which you can respond to life's situations with equanimity.

A Deeper Exploration: Two Elegant Meanings of "Tree Pose"

On its face, Tree Pose's Sanskrit name is very clear and descriptive—it is *Vrskasana*, with *vrska* (pronounced "vrick-sha") meaning a tree or the trunk of a tree, and *asana* meaning posture. But my favorite translation says that the pose refers to "any tree bearing visible flowers and fruit."[5] When you practice Tree Pose, you might like to imagine your center like the trunk of a tree, rooted strongly enough to withstand whatever winds may come your way and to be resilient in the face of life's emotional storms. In this image, your outstretched arms become the flowers or fruit that blossom on your firmly grounded tree trunk. What will bloom in you today?

Another image associated with Tree Pose is an eight-petaled lotus flower that, according to yoga tradition, resides in your fourth *chakra*, your heart center. When the energy of the heart center is "closed," the lotus flower is sealed shut. As you reach upward and lift your arms, like branches growing toward sunlight, visualize the lotus flower in your heart center opening and coming into full bloom.

5. Restorative Bridge Pose I (with a Bolster)

Now that you've moved your body both physically and energetically, you'll practice a restorative backbend to help release any tension in your abdomen and diaphragm while gently opening your chest and heart.

Honestly, gently, and openly facing our emotions—and giving them a pathway toward healthy expression—is our goal in this pose. Restorative Bridge Pose I helps to open your chest and diaphragm, which can help you breathe more fully and release tension. Remaining in a supported position like Restorative Bridge Pose I for even a few minutes can help bring your mind into a centered, focused state, which helps ground you in the present moment. As the well-known trauma expert Bessel van der Kolk, MD, has discovered in years of research on the effect of yoga on trauma survivors, "Simply noticing what you feel fosters emotional regulation, and it helps you to stop trying to ignore what is going on inside you."[6]

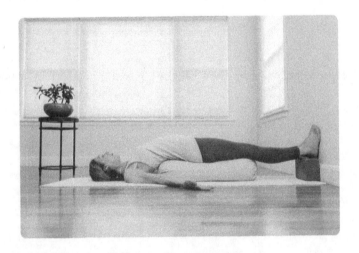

Place your mat with its short end against a wall, and place a bolster or three folded blankets perpendicular to the wall, about eighteen inches from it. Place a block against the wall in either the "medium" or "high" position. Sit on the bolster facing the wall with your feet firmly on the floor. Slowly lie back on the bolster and move your body back until your shoulders and head are resting on the floor. Place your heels on the block with the soles of your feet grounded into the wall. Your legs should be straight. It may take several adjustments before you find the best placement for the bolster relative to the wall. Rest your arms on the floor with your palms facing toward the ceiling.

Once you've found the right place for your bolster, take a few moments to scan your body and make sure it's comfortable. Your lower back needs to be completely at ease—if you feel compression or discomfort in your back, try using one or two folded blankets instead of a bolster for a less intense backbend. If your knees aren't supported by your blankets or bolster, place a folded blanket or block underneath them. Your goal is to feel complete relaxation throughout your body.

Notice the pattern and quality of your breath in Restorative Bridge Pose I. As your body relaxes and your chest opens, focus on making your exhalations full and long. When you change your breathing pattern, you can bring balance to your nervous system. You may feel a shift in your emotions; Dr. Streeter's research shows that much of the difference in reported feelings of anger, sadness, fear, and joy can be connected to the ways in which we control our breath.[7] The energetic process of using breath to regulate your nervous system is central—if you'll forgive the pun—to the centering journey we are undertaking in this chapter.

Remain in Restorative Bridge Pose I for about five minutes, or as long as your mind can pay attention to your internal sensations. When you are ready to come out of the pose, bend your knees, roll over onto one side of your body, and then sit up. Sit with your eyes closed for a few moments and try to maintain the open sensation in your chest. Remember—your open chest is a doorway to your inner self, a pathway for your mind to travel toward your center.

6. Child's Pose—Side Stretch Variation

After practicing a backbend, it is appropriate to equalize the extension of the spinal muscles with a forward bend, which brings flexion and length to the spine. It is important to respect your spine by mindfully transitioning from a backbend to a forward bend, lengthening your spinal muscles so they have time to return to a neutral position before you fold forward. You'll make that transition here with a variation of Child's Pose that elongates the spine and trunk before you come into Supported Child's Pose Forward Bend as the next step in the exploration of your center.

Sit with your knees bent and your hips nestled onto your feet. If your hips don't reach your feet, place a folded blanket or bolster between your calves and the backs of your thighs. Your knees should be about one foot apart. Inhale, lift up through your trunk, and raise your arms over your head. As you exhale, bend forward at your hips and extend your arms, waist, and chest forward. Rest your forehead on the floor. If your head doesn't reach the floor, support it on a block. In this first stage of Child's

Pose, you are actively elongating your torso forward, allowing your lower back muscles to return to their natural length. You'll know you're doing this correctly if you can feel your abdomen and front ribs lengthening as they rest against your thighs. With your breath soft and normal, stay in this stretch for fifteen to twenty seconds.

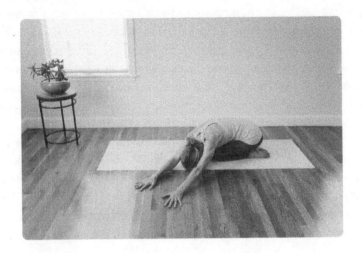

Now lift your head and trunk, turn to the left, place your hands to the left of your left leg, and fold your trunk down to rest on your thigh. Reach your right arm actively away from your hips so you feel length all along the right side of your body, from your hip through your armpit. Stay here for a few long, deep breaths, and then lift halfway up and repeat the pose on your right side. After remaining on that side for an equal number of breaths, come back to the starting point with your trunk centered on your legs, then draw your hands toward your body to help lift yourself upward.

7. Supported Child's Pose Forward Bend

Place a bolster or three folded blankets between your knees (but not so far back that they extend under your hips). If you have problems with your knees, place a folded blanket behind them. Fold your trunk forward from your hip joints, allowing your spine to gently round, and bring your abdomen and chest to rest on the bolster or blankets. If your abdomen doesn't reach the bolster or if your head isn't relaxed, add more height under your trunk. Take a moment to observe your body and feel whether it's completely comfortable—it needs to be if you are going to enjoy the pose. The intention of a supported seated forward bend is to be so comfortable that your back body can release muscular tension and your mind can become quiet.

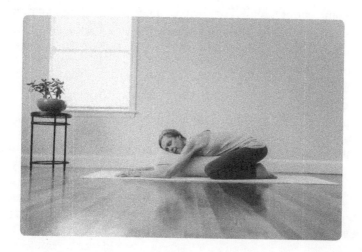

Imagine your spine elegantly draped over your body, a string of perfect pearls that traces your body's long, beautiful center. Draw your attention to the beginning of the string of pearls at the base of your spine, the first *chakra*, your root *chakra*, your center of groundedness. Breathe into it and feel yourself rooted to the earth. With each inhale, draw your attention up along the string of pearls and imagine the brilliant, luminous energy that exists at each of your six other *chakras*:

Second *chakra*: Your sacrum; the center of creativity
Third *chakra*: Behind your navel; the center of personal power
Fourth *chakra*: Behind your heart; the center of emotions
Fifth *chakra*: Behind your throat; the center of self-expression
Sixth *chakra*: In the center of your skull; the center of inner wisdom
Seventh *chakra*: The crown of your head; the center of universal connection

Now it's time to turn your attention inward, toward your deep and rich energetic center. Close your eyes if they aren't already closed. If that's not comfortable for you, close your eyes halfway. In this head-down position with less external stimuli, your eyes have an opportunity to let go of looking outward, and your attention can "look" within. Imagine your ears could listen inwardly, to your deepest and most sincere thoughts. In that scenario, you would begin to experience the withdrawal of your sense organs, a yoga practice called *pratyahara*.

Slowly come out of Child's Pose by pressing your hands into your mat so that your trunk comes up lightly, without overexerting your back muscles. Sit back on your hips and stretch your legs straight out in front of you. Check in with yourself, honoring your feelings and thoughts.

A Deeper Exploration: Drawing the Senses Inward (*Pratyahara*)

Our sense organs—including our eyes, ears, and skin—tell us so much about the world around us. But sometimes it's calming and healing to take a break from the outside world, and refocus on the universe of sensations inside our bodies. In yoga philosophy, this process is called *pratyahara*, which means "withdrawal of the senses."[8] This term appears in the **Yoga Sutras of Patañjali**, a central philosophical sourcebook for yoga practice that I mentioned earlier in this book. To show you how important *pratyahara* is, it is named as one of eight "limbs" of yoga practice (the other limbs include postures—*asana*—and breath work—*pranayama*). In *pratyahara*, your sense organs are freed from the push and pull of everyday concerns. You may still notice external occurrences like sounds or the temperature of a room, but those sensations do not penetrate your state of peaceful rest. You are aware of them, but not disturbed by them. Your sense organs turn inward, as if they could see, listen to, and feel the deep inner peace that exists in your center.

8. Centering Inverted Pose

Inverted postures like this one hold an important place in managing depression and anxiety.

Here's why—when you lie down with your legs supported by a wall and a bolster or folded blankets under your hips, your body rests in a gentle, supported backbend, similar to but even more powerful than what you practiced earlier in Restorative Bridge Pose I. In Inverted Pose, yogically speaking, the energy of your legs flows down and pools in your lower abdomen and then flows softly from your abdomen into your chest, bathing the heart. Your chest and heart areas open and broaden, and your breath deepens. As in Restorative Bridge Pose I, you may find that your exhalations can become smooth and long during Inverted Pose, promoting profound relaxation throughout your nervous system.

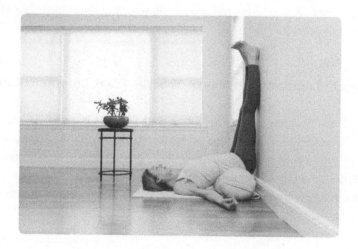

To come into Inverted Pose, sit with one side of your body at a wall, with a bolster or folded blankets nearby. Turn your trunk and head away from the wall while you lift your legs vertically up the wall. Take a few moments to adjust your body so that it is square to the wall, then bend your knees and place the soles of your feet on the wall. Lift your hips, slide your bolster or blankets under your hips, and rest your hips comfortably on the props. You know you're in the pose correctly if your lower abdomen is flat and your chest is in a gentle backbend. If your lower abdomen is tilted upward, try using less height under your hips, and be sure to press your shoulders gently down into the earth to broaden your upper chest.

Once you are comfortable, close your eyes and allow your attention to focus on your chest. Envision the journey toward your center—specifically, visualize your heart center, or *Anahata chakra*, residing behind your physical heart in the center of your spine. According to some of the earliest written texts of the yoga traditions, the heart center is the source of our very essence as well as a place of joy and peace.[9]

Imagine these qualities in your heart center. I hope that, once you experience even a glimpse of this energy, you will understand that it is always present for you and accessible to you, especially in times of deepest need. When you are dispirited from depression, feeling isolated, disconnected, and alone, you can remind yourself of this connection to something stable and strong in your center. When you are nervous, restless, or overwrought, it can be an oasis of calming energy.

Remain in Inverted Pose for about five minutes. When you are ready to come out of the pose, bend your knees and roll to one side, and then slowly lift your trunk and sit for a few moments in any comfortable seated position.

9. Deep Relaxation with Ocean Breath—Your Luminous Center

Resting in Deep Relaxation at the end of a yoga practice is a pose as important as any other. This precious gift of time allows the benefits of yoga to seep into your cells. This experience can lead to reduced levels of anxiety and stress and increased levels of self-awareness, compassion, and introspection, each of which is a tool for self-understanding and self-acceptance, important final steps on the journey toward your peaceful center.[10]

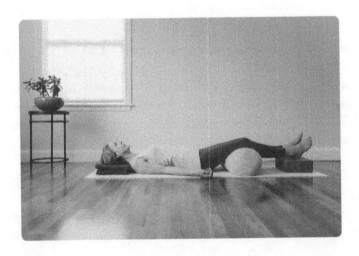

So that you rest in complete comfort, I suggest placing a folded blanket under your head and a bolster under your knees. If you are comfortable using an eye pillow, you'll find it gently reminds the area around your eyes to relax, and directs your attention away from the everyday world. If you are feeling ungrounded or unstable, lie down with your feet resting against a wall, place a block under each foot (pictured), or nestle a folded blanket against each outer thigh.

Once your body feels settled and comfortable, pay attention to your inner world. Feel your inhale as it moves down into your body from your nose to your feet, and feel grounded to the earth. As you exhale, feel your breath moving from your feet all the way to the crown of your head, and feel lightness and softness in your head, as if your brain itself were relaxing. Visualize your breath as a light that flows through the center of your body like a wave, an ebb and flow of luminous, enriching, life-affirming energy.

As your breath deepens, let it direct your attention once again to your heart center, *Anahata chakra*, the literal center of your energetic body. As you rest, you can explore this *chakra* a little more deeply. The Sanskrit word *Anahata* means "unstruck" or "unwounded, intact."[11] Imagine the purity and clarity of this inner place that hasn't been touched or changed by your emotional experiences! One of my favorite descriptions of the energy of the heart center is "shimmering emptiness that is the source of this world."[12] Remember our discussion of the two meanings of center? *Anahata chakra* meets both definitions—it is the energetic center of your body, and it is also a transcendent source, larger than your life experiences and abounding with pure joy, peace, and the energy of your essential Self.

With this imagery in mind, visualize energy shimmering through your body into your heart center. You might like to imagine it as a soothing, iridescent shade of green, the color of the heart *chakra* in yogic mythology. Visualize an expansive, verdant space where you can cultivate peace, tranquility, and composure. With each inhale, imagine your inner field of tranquility growing outward, enveloping your body in calmness, and with each exhale feel your mind becoming more centered.

A farmer plants seeds, watches over fields, tends to plants with attention and loving care, and sees her effort come to fruition when the harvest arrives. As you practice yoga, you too are developing tools to sow seeds of centeredness in the verdant field of your heart. Tend to your field with love, and you will feel your center grow and blossom.

Now that you've glimpsed the beautiful, shimmering energy of your heart center and felt how it can soothe your mind and emotions, perhaps your sense organs can turn inward and "contentedly dwell within."[13] Perhaps your attention can rest deeply in your heart, in peaceful respite from the thoughts and feelings that usually occupy it. In this centered state, you will find that your emotions lose their charge and become more manageable, and your heart and mind will feel clarity and peace.

Now you will bring Ocean Breath, the practice we started with, into your Deep Relaxation. As you exhale, gently, softly, and slightly contract the back of your throat until you hear the soft vibration of your breath. Feel your normal, long inhale lifting up through your body from the base of your spine into your heart, and feel your Ocean Breath exhale flowing out from your heart, down to the base of your spine. If you feel very comfortable with Ocean Breath, you can practice using it to breathe both in and out. If you struggle with Ocean Breath at any time, let go of it, and move onward to your Coherent Breathing practice.

After five or six rounds of Ocean Breath, take a few normal breaths and then transition into your twenty-minute Coherent Breathing practice, which I described in Chapter 4. To practice Coherent Breathing, have your timer or Coherent Breathing app set to five breaths per minute (a six-second inhalation and a six-second exhalation).

After you've finished your Coherent Breathing practice, remain in Deep Relaxation as long as your body is comfortable and your mind stays present to your inner feelings. To come out, slowly move your extremities, roll over onto your side, and ease yourself into a comfortable seated position.

Observe how your intention to practice yoga in a state of centeredness has changed your mind—and perhaps changed your answers to the three questions you asked yourself before your practice:

1. Where is your center? Do you feel more connected to it?
2. Are you able to get a glimpse of your true self at your center?
3. What one word, feeling, or image comes to mind following your practice?

Perhaps you are experiencing less negative self-talk, the kind that holds you back from living your life fully, or perhaps your thoughts are less frenetic, with space and silence around them. You have taken a journey within and you have found your center, a place you can return to whenever you need support. Now, you are connected to yourself.

CHAPTER 6

EMPOWER

Inner strength fuels the journey toward your fullest life.

How strong are you? How much faith do you have in your power to thrive in your everyday life?

In an ideal world, your answer would be a confident "I am super-strong!" You would believe in your ability to meet the responsibilities of your everyday life, trust that you have a source of wellness and peace within your body and mind, and feel motivated to do great things each and every day.

When you are struggling under the weight of depression or feel frozen by anxiety, though, your answer might be distant and unsatisfying. "I used to be stronger," you might say. Or, "I wish I had more inner strength."

Healing emotionally requires strength and confidence—two things that can feel out of reach when your moods are imbalanced. But when you make time to practice yoga, even if it's just two or three times each week, you will cultivate an inner strength that becomes a reservoir of empowerment that will help support your everyday life. Without any fear of failure, you can begin to feel free to become your fully empowered self.

Melanie, who participated in our study, is a wonderful example of how yoga helps build inner strength. A recent college graduate, she had been looking for employment for six months in her high-tech field, but she was having no luck. She wanted to find a job in Chicago, where her family lives, even though the jobs she was most interested in were highly competitive. Melanie would often arrive for yoga sessions having just received yet another job rejection, which added a destabilizing layer of anxiety to her general stress and lack of self-confidence.

It amazes me how often the physical work of yoga practice maps cleanly onto a practitioner's personal journey. This was particularly true for Melanie. As our work together progressed, I watched as she connected with an inner strength that gave her the confidence to be stable in both her thoughts and her poses. I started to notice a shift in Melanie, from having difficulty finding stability, both in her overly flexible body and in her overactive mind, to becoming more physically grounded, stronger, and mentally focused.

That inner strength helped Melanie make an important life choice. At her last session, she announced that she had received a job offer. But the position was in a smaller city in a different state, so she decided not to accept it. She shared that she now realized she was employable, had valuable skills to offer, and was confident enough to hold out for the right job in the right city. Her statement both stunned and delighted me. It was a beautiful realization of her self-worth—a display of the inner strength required to take her future into her own hands—to act in her best self-interest.

The stability and grounding she gained through yoga practice had a big part in Melanie's mental and emotional shift. Let's explore how accessing your inner strength can do the same for you.

WHAT IS EMPOWERMENT?

Yoga philosophy encourages us to be active participants in our own lives, for it is through participation that we learn the tools for becoming our best selves. This philosophy is stated plainly in the first-century text the *Bhagavad Gita*, which says, "Know what your duty is, and do it without hesitation."[1] If that isn't the definition of confidence, I don't know what is!

The poetic *Gita*, which is an important part of yogic philosophy, is a dramatic story that takes the form of a dialogue between Krishna, who turns out to be a divine figure in disguise, and Arjuna, a reluctant warrior who has dropped his weapons and refused to fight in a battle against his cousins. To shore up Arjuna's resolve, inner strength, and personal power, Krishna further counsels the young man to do his duty, "without concern for results."[2] To be successful in life, the *Gita* teaches, we must feel empowered to discover our own path and travel confidently on it, without attachment to a particular outcome or result.

This might sound like an oxymoron. After all, aren't strong people the ones who accomplish their life's goals? Doesn't empowerment go hand in hand with success?

According to yoga philosophy, the simple answer is, "Not always." In the yogic view, inner strength comes from having the courage to act, not from having each action bring us success and accomplishment. Engaging fully with your life—in times of joy as well as challenge—is the goal of empowerment. As Krishna assures Arjuna in the *Bhagavad Gita*, "On this path no effort is wasted."[3]

HOW EMPOWERMENT HELPS EASE
DEPRESSION AND ANXIETY

When you are mired in a depressive episode or anxious thought-swirl, it can feel intimidating to be asked to find your source of inner strength and empowerment. But connecting with this grounded confidence is a crucial component of healing emotionally. Becoming empowered is not an accomplishment—it is an ever-present state of emotional well-being, one that will accompany you on any journey you endeavor to take in your life. There will be times when being empowered means valuing yourself enough to say "no" to an opportunity that's not quite right for you, as Melanie did. And there will be times when facing a challenge with confidence—as Arjuna did—becomes more important than achieving victory over that challenge.

Empowerment can be a beacon of hope when depression whispers that you are neither strong nor skilled enough to live your fullest life. It can also quiet an anxious mind that is too afraid of failure to try new things or confront uncomfortable issues.

As you work toward finding your life path, you will find the power and inner strength to act in the world. And by cultivating an attitude that helps you let go of the results of your actions, you will release the anxiety that comes with worrying about the future, as well as the depressive ruminations about past events that you feel were not your best moments. Empowerment enables you to be free of both the past and the future, which leaves you firmly grounded in each present moment. This is exactly where you need to be to feel the sensations in your body and listen to the thoughts in your mind and heart.

BRING YOUR HEART INTO THE PRESENT MOMENT

Our empowering practice will connect you with the sort of inner strength I've been describing—confident, awake, and driven toward a positive, engaged life, but not determined to achieve any particular definition of "success." The empowerment we are after is not an athletic endeavor or a physical accomplishment you will either achieve or not. Instead, this practice will help you connect with the strength you need to find the present moment and dwell there in a state of energetic peace.

Before we begin, we'll do a simple exercise to come into the present moment. Sit comfortably with your spine tall, your chest soft and open, and your eyes halfway or fully closed. Draw your mind into your heart band, the area of your chest that surrounds your heart center. As you learned in Chapter 5, the heart center is the home of your emotions. As you breathe in a natural rhythm, pay attention for the inner messages and deepest desires your heart wants to share with you. Focus on becoming present to each moment, letting go of the previous moment and not worrying about what's to come. As you concentrate on your heart center, feel its intense power, its role as a source of inner strength that strives to create a good and balanced life for you. Let it do its work. Feel the personal power you hold in this present moment. After several breaths, open your eyes and get ready for your empowering yoga practice.

THREE QUESTIONS TO PREPARE YOU FOR PRACTICE

Before you begin this yoga sequence, ask yourself these three questions. Note your reactions in an open-minded, nonjudgmental way. There are no wrong answers!

1. How do you define inner strength for yourself?
2. What activities in your daily life make you feel the most powerful?
3. When you bring your attention to your heart center, how does it feel? Open? Tight? Strong? Quiet?

Turn the page to begin your practice. And remember, staying present to yourself from moment to moment, accessing your inner strength, and acting from a place of personal power will help to calm your mind when it needs soothing and inspire you to get up and live your life when you feel depressed. I chose poses for this empower-ment practice that will help you cultivate these qualities—presence of mind, inner strength, and profound power. They will help you to become empowered from the inside, and they will give you tools to bring your empowerment out into the world, to create the best life possible for yourself.

YOGA PRACTICE FOR EMPOWERMENT

1. Cross-Legged Seated Pose with Ocean Breath

Sit comfortably with your legs crossed on the floor or on a folded blanket, or sit in a chair if you prefer. Your spine should lift upward and your chest should be broad and open. Close your eyes halfway or all the way, and take a couple of minutes to notice the thoughts that come into your mind. Are they positive and constructive, or are they self-defeating? Do they encourage you to face your day or to run away from it? Pay attention to each thought as it comes, and to the emotions that rise up to meet it. You don't need to act on your emotions yet; just observe and acknowledge them as you remember that all emotions are valid if they can be catalysts for action.

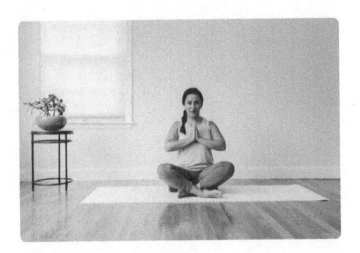

Bring your hands into Prayer Position by placing your palms together in front of your heart. Create an intention for your practice; visualize yourself finding a sense of personal empowerment, whatever that might look like for you. Identify any self-defeating thought that arises, and now, as I described in Chapter 2, change it into a positive thought by cultivating an opposite feeling. Remember that we become empowered little by little, changing our feelings of insecurity into self-worth, transforming our worries and concerns into constructive actions. Release your hands and gently rest them on your thighs in the Gesture of Consciousness.

Quiet your mind with two to three minutes of Ocean Breath, inhaling normally and then gently contracting your throat muscles to create a full, resonant Ocean Breath exhale. For this empowering practice, if you are comfortable, create the same "inner sigh" sound for your inhalations and exhalations, visualizing the quality of inner strength materializing with each breath. As you inhale, picture a strong flow of life force moving into your entire body, enlivening and awakening even its smallest parts, so your body becomes a vehicle for moving forward into self-empowerment. As you exhale, practice letting go of the results of each breath, and feel each one creating peace in your mind.

2. Hero's Pose with Upward Bound Knuckle Pose

Hero's Pose stimulates the energy of the legs, hips, and arms—the very places in your body that help you move through your day with purpose and clarity. Especially if you're feeling lethargic from depression or if your mind is overactive with anxiety, paying attention to these centers of movement is an empowering experience. And, it has the added value of having a name that might inspire you to own some of the heroic qualities you discover within yourself!

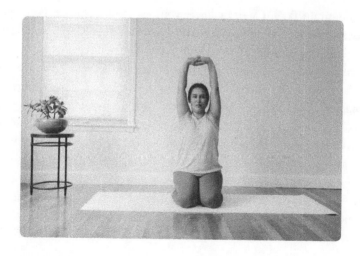

Come onto your hands and knees, turn your toes in and your heels out, and sit down on your heels. If this is uncomfortable for your ankles or knees, move your feet away from each other, place a block or a stack of blocks horizontally between your feet, and sit on the blocks. Alternatively, sit comfortably in a chair. Close or lower your eyes. Breathe down into your lower belly. Visualize your root *chakra* connecting with the earth, and feel how the floor or the seat of your chair grounds and supports your body. Keep breathing into your lower belly, and now visualize your sacral *chakra*, your center of creativity, becoming stimulated and alive.

Interlace your fingers. Turn your palms forward and lift your arms straight up in Upward Bound Knuckle Pose. Take two or three breaths, reaching up with every part of your arms and pressing your palms toward the sky. Keep your head in a neutral position and gaze softly forward. Bring your arms down, reverse the interlace of your fingers, and repeat the pose.

When you are done, sit quietly for a moment and feel your legs, hips, and arms alive and energized, ready to help you get up and go. Meditate on the qualities of a hero—he is self-confident yet grounded, courageous, and focused; she meets adversity with creativity, flexibility, and inner strength. As you breathe, visualize these qualities within yourself.

3. Empowering Sun Salutation

Stand in Mountain Pose. Close or lower your eyes and meditate momentarily on the qualities of the sun, which powers our planet. It gives us light and heat. It creates energy and life. Without it, we simply would not be alive.

Practice two rounds of Sun Salutation, now turning your focus to your inner sun, your fiery third *chakra* that powers your whole being. This energy center—called *Manipura chakra* in Sanskrit—is located within the spine between your navel and your solar plexus. Breathe into it, visualizing the flow of life force igniting the power of your inner sun. Each time you exhale, visualize this power moving completely through your body. Feel the heat and light of your sun, your source of energy and light, empowering you to move out into the world and proceed with all that lies before you. Feel confident that you can inhabit each day from a place of inner strength and personal empowerment. When you are finished and back in Mountain Pose, close or lower your eyes and feel how this dynamic flow has shifted your energy level. It's no coincidence that the third *chakra* is recognized as your center of personal power. After practicing Sun Salutation, enjoy the sense of self-confidence from strengthening and opening your body. Perhaps you feel empowered to move more strongly and energetically through your day.

See pages 172–173 for a photographic Sun Salutation refresher.
> *Mountain Pose*
> *Upward Hand Pose*
> *Standing Forward Bend Pose*
> *Standing Forward Bend Pose—Head Up*
> *Standing Forward Bend Pose*
> *Downward Facing Dog Pose*
> *High Plank Pose*
> *Four Limb Staff Pose*
> *Cobra Pose or Upward Facing Dog Pose*
> *Downward Facing Dog Pose*
> *Standing Forward Bend Pose*
> *Standing Forward Bend Pose—Head Up*
> *Standing Forward Bend Pose*
> *Upward Hand Pose*
> *Mountain Pose*

4. Warrior I

Now that you've contemplated your inner hero and awakened your inner sun, it's time to power up your body with Warrior I, a robust standing pose that helps awaken and strengthen your legs, hips, and abdominal core. Your spine is elongated and your heart will be lifted, both physically and metaphorically speaking, in this pose. Warrior I will teach you to meet the world with the courage and fierceness of a warrior—a warrior who is dedicated to healing the heart and mind.

Stand in Mountain Pose and step your feet four feet apart. Turn your left foot in about 45 degrees, and turn your right foot out 90 degrees. Turn your trunk so that your hips and trunk are facing forward, over your right leg. Inhale deeply while you raise your arms over your head, and exhale as you bend your right knee

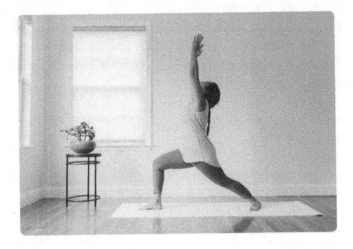

and "sit down" into the pose. Glance at your right knee—it should be directly over your ankle—and then gaze straight forward, or if you feel strong and balanced, look up toward the sky. Stay in the pose for a few breaths. With each inhale, reach strongly from your feet up through your trunk and arms, and with each exhale, find your foundation as energy flows through your body into the earth. Straighten your front leg to come out of the pose as you inhale. Turn your feet so they are parallel with each other, and step them together, returning to Mountain Pose. Now practice the pose on your opposite side.

5. Supported Reclining Backbend Pose

In Chapter 4, I talked about how backbends are useful for depression because they open the heart in both physical and emotional ways. I think of them as tools to break down body armor, the layers of self-protection that accumulate from stressful or traumatic experiences. When your body armor cracks and falls away, the intuitive wisdom of your heart, and your true nature, are revealed.

Sit on your mat with two blocks within reach. Place one block in the "medium" height position horizontally across your mat, and place the other block in the "high" position a few inches behind the first one. Sit with your back to the

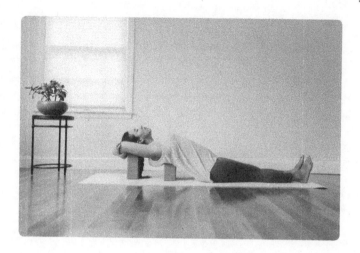

blocks, with your knees bent and your hips eight to ten inches in front of the blocks. Hold the first block—the "medium" one—with your hands and slowly lie back, bringing your shoulder blades onto the block so it supports your heart band. Place your head on the second, "high" block. Take a few moments to adjust your body so you are comfortable. You can turn your blocks up or down to adjust the pose for more or less stretch. Let your arms rest by your sides, palms up, or hold your elbows and rest your forearms on your forehead or gently against the crown of your head.

Breathe into the center of your heart area and visualize the empowering energy that lives there. Is it brilliantly bright, drawing your inner light outward for the world to behold? Perhaps it feels just the opposite—heavy and dark, as if enclosed by layers of opaqueness that dim its light. Remember during the dark times that even though the light is covered up, it is still there. Use each inhalation to feel your heart area expanding by any amount possible. As you exhale, feel the area around your heart softening, releasing tension and emotion away from your heart center, allowing the radiant light of your true nature to slowly but surely shine through.

Stay in the pose for five minutes, or longer if it feels comfortable and restful. To come out, place your hands palms-down on the floor, and press your trunk up to a seated position.

A Deeper Exploration: Your True Nature

You discovered *Anahata chakra*, or the heart center, in Chapter 5, when we discussed this *chakra* as the literal center of your energetic body. This *chakra* also has a lot to teach us about our personal power. In the yogic traditions, there is a seed of cosmic energy that lives within each of us at the heart center. Take a moment to consider this expansive idea—the energy in *Anahata chakra* is the same energy that makes up the entire cosmos. It is boundless, unchanging, pure, and whole. Because it dwells in your heart center, this cosmic energy is, in fact, your true nature, your true "Self." It unites you with the cosmos and each being in it; we are all made of this energy. Each time you practice a backbend, finding and opening your heart, you have an opportunity to remember the energy of your true nature. Think of it as stable, present, and always available to you. It is a wellspring of support that can empower you to take an action when you are depressed, or to remind you to slow your mind down and rest in your heart when you are anxious.

6. Reclining Bent Knee Twist

Now, you'll release your spinal muscles and any tension in your back with a gentle twist, to soothe and relax your body before you transition into a forward bend. Lie

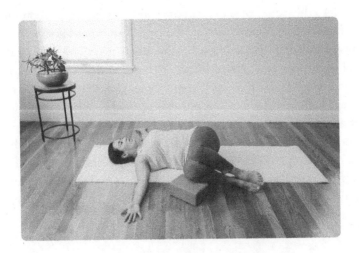

down on your back with your knees bent and your feet firmly placed on the floor. Stretch your arms straight out along the floor, forming a right angle at your shoulders. One by one, bring your knees into your chest. Inhale deeply, and take your knees over to your right as you exhale. Linger here, taking a few breaths and adjusting your legs so you are in a comfortable, soft twist. You can take your legs over to the right as far as is comfortable, but be sure your left shoulder remains on the floor. You may like to place a block under your right thigh to ease the twist.

You should feel length and release along your spinal muscles. As you relax into the pose, visualize tension draining away, your body becoming quiet. Your heart band should feel broad and open, as you visualize the abiding and healing energy of your heart center spreading outward through your body, supporting and empowering you onward in your life.

Come out of the pose by drawing your knees up toward your right shoulder and then over to the center of your body, before repeating the pose on the opposite side.

7. Head-to-Knee Pose

Now you'll practice a seated pose that will draw you a little more deeply into a forward bend than the Child's Pose you practiced in Chapter 5. Head-to-Knee Pose stretches the legs and spine and opens the hips. As with all forward bends, it also stimulates the energy of the abdomen. In yoga philosophy, the abdomen—the upper and lower belly—is considered to be in charge of digestion, the absorption of nutrients, elimination, and the discharge of toxins. Since yoga practice encompasses the entire body and mind, our focus is not only on digesting and absorbing food but also on digesting and absorbing—or processing—emotions as well.

Sit on your mat with your legs straight out in front of you, with one or two blocks within reach. If your legs feel tight, have a belt nearby. Stay here for a few breaths, feeling your legs and hips well-grounded, and your spine lifting. Your spinal muscles should feel active but not strained; if you can't lift your chest, sit up on a folded blanket. Bend your left knee and place your left foot along the inside of your right thigh, with your left knee relaxing down toward the floor. Lift your arms overhead, and as you exhale, fold forward from your hips until you can hold your right foot with your hand or belt. Keeping both your abdomen and neck long, gaze down toward your right leg.

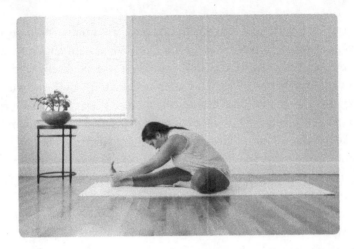

Check in with yourself. How do you feel, both physically and mentally? If your body feels discomfort or if your mind feels stressed, bend your right knee and hold your right foot with your belt. Remain in this stage for a few breaths, continuing to monitor yourself. When you've found a comfortable position, support your forehead on your blocks, letting go of any tension in your neck and letting your brain and eyes become quiet.

Breathe into your belly, and as you exhale, visualize any unhelpful or unnecessary tension releasing from your body into the earth and flowing away. Breathe out any self-limiting thoughts and emotions. Breath by breath, visualize your body, heart, and mind becoming cleansed and clear. You've activated the energy of your abdomen, and it is purifying your whole self. You have made room for new thoughts and emotions, for the quality of self-empowerment to fill the spaces that self-defeat and self-limitation no longer inhabit.

Come out of this pose by gently looking forward and then raising your arms and trunk upward. Change legs, and repeat on the opposite side.

8. Empowering Inverted Pose

Part of being empowered is having the courage to let go and come into a state of true rest. Give yourself permission to rest now in a supported, inverted backbend.

This might seem quite different from the kind of empowerment that I've described so far, but it is the other side of the coin, so to speak. Taking the time to rest, to take no action, will help quiet your body, mind, and senses. Your chest will gently open, your breath will become soft and deep, and the story of your heart's desires can become clear. Remember that Melanie became empowered when she gave herself permission to turn down a job she intuitively knew wasn't right for her. She listened to her heart and acted to support her deepest desires. In this practice of Inverted Pose, there is no work to do but to enjoy resting and listening to your inner self.

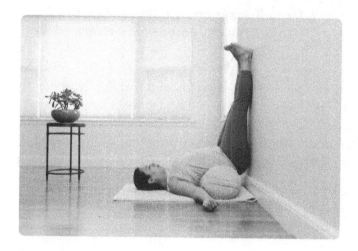

Sit with your side body next to a wall, lie down, and swing your legs up the wall. Slide a bolster under your hips to come into Inverted Pose. Once you are up, briefly scan your body, especially your hips and back, to make sure you are in a state of complete comfort. Otherwise, take time to change the height of the props under your hips. You can lift your hips higher by adding a blanket, or lower them by using less support. The important thing is that your body can rest deeply without being distracted by any physical discomfort.

In Inverted Pose, feel the soft vibration of your breath and life force as it flows from your legs down into your belly, and then softly into your heart, where it gathers and settles. Experience your chest as spacious, almost limitless, and feel the power within it as pure, transcendent, and infinite. You have cracked the armor of your outer body—the layers of your chest are open. Let the messages of your heart come from the darkness into the light.

Remain in Inverted Pose for five minutes. When you are ready to come out, bend your knees and roll over onto your side. Take a few breaths to release your back, and slowly come to a seated position. Sit with your eyes lowered or closed for a few moments to appreciate the messages that have made their way from your heart to your mind.

9. Deep Relaxation with Ocean Breath— Your Brilliant, Empowered Heart

In this practice, you've broken through some layers of overly protective body armor and discarded some of the dark coverings that may have been surrounding your heart and holding you back from accessing your inner strength. You have let in the light, and your heart is now empowered to share its truth with you. Resting in Deep Relaxation will give you some quality time with this newfound—or enhanced—sense of personal power, allowing it to permeate every cell in your body.

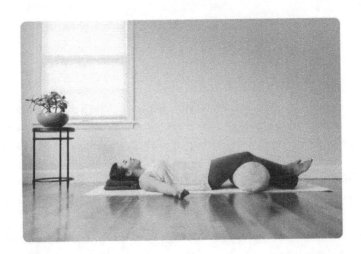

Lie down with a bolster or folded blanket under your thighs and your head supported on a blanket. Gently bow to the wisdom of your heart with a gentle nod of the chin toward your chest. Cover yourself with a blanket, if you'd like, and place an eye pillow across your eyes for extra comfort. Rest your feet on a rolled-up blanket if that appeals to you. You'll be lying down for almost twenty minutes, so be sure your body is happy. Of course, you can change your position at any time.

Once you are comfortable, reflect on the light you have cultivated within yourself, starting in Sun Salutation and building throughout this empowering practice. The image of this powerful light takes us back to the *Bhagavad Gita*, the text where we began our empowering journey. As the deity Krishna reveals his true form to the warrior Arjuna in the story, we read, "If a thousand suns were to rise and stand in the noon sky, blazing, such brilliance would be like the fierce brilliance of that mighty Self."[4] Having completed this practice, can you feel your point of connection with this vast, cosmic energy? Do you feel your own inner sun as, perhaps, one of a thousand that illuminates your world, your life?

When you are ready, inhale normally, gently contract your throat, and practice five to six rounds of Ocean Breath. Maintain the image of the brilliant light of empowerment collecting in your heart center as you inhale and diffusing through your entire body as you exhale. Let the light warm you, soothe you, and empower you.

Finish your Ocean Breath and take a few normal breaths as you prepare to transition into Coherent Breathing. During this twenty-minute practice, just let the even flow of your breath do its work, infusing your entire being with the brilliance of your empowering inner light.

You might like to return to the questions you brought into your practice, checking in with yourself to see if you have fresh insights on your personal power.

1. Do you have a new perspective on what inner strength feels like to you?
2. At what point in the practice did you feel the most powerful?
3. Bring your attention to your heart center once more. How does it feel?

You are now ready to bring this sense of peaceful, luminous strength into the rest of your day—and into every day after.

CHAPTER 7

ENERGIZE

Activate your body and mind;
let your passion awaken.

To live well, we need the get-up-and-go to inspire us to move. But to get out of bed in the morning feeling fresh and ready to meet the day can seem like a Herculean task when depression slows our bodies. The endurance to make it through the day with a clear mind can feel like an unattainable goal when we are sapped of the vital energy we need to be fully awake in the world. Depression can make us feel trapped and sluggish.

Activating your body and mind means releasing the "stuck" places inside and inviting fresh, vibrant energy back into your life. When something is clogged—a gutter, a vacuum cleaner bag, even a human artery—it has to work harder to fulfill its purpose. The rain drips slowly through the pressed leaves that block the gutter; the vacuum cleaner engine whirs and whines to make its dusty collection; the artery throbs blood through the body with great effort. When these passages are clear, though, when they become unstuck, they perform with ease, power, and efficiency. Their energy flows without excessive exertion.

So can yours.

This chapter will give you helpful tools to help awaken your vital inner energy and meet each day feeling eager and alive.

WHAT IS YOUR ENERGY SOURCE?

On a day-to-day basis, energy comes from taking care of your body and mind and living a healthy life. We could talk at length about the roles that the right nutrition, hydration, sleep, and movement play in contributing to our overall energy levels.

But I want to focus our attention on another kind of vital energy, a more fundamental source of vigor that exists in a deeper place than our refrigerators, beds, and gyms—something yoga philosophers refer to as the "energetic body." Yoga philosophy posits that there are five "bodies" or "layers" to each person's being. Second only to the physical layer is the energetic layer, which reflects how fundamental to our functioning this layer is. Without sufficient energy, our minds, bodies, and spirits simply don't have enough fuel.

From earlier discussions in this book, you probably remember the definition of the yogic concept of *prana* as "life force." Another definition is "vital energy."[1] In the yogic view of the body, *prana* is a dynamic and unending flow of life-sustaining vitality. Just as you know when your energy level is vibrant and awake or, literally, depressed, you can feel the presence—or dearth—of *prana* in your body. The subtle variation of your breath will tell you when *prana* is flowing in an unrestricted way or when it is depleted, blocked, or stuck. Although Sanskrit can sometimes sound complicated to Western ears, you will recognize *prana* in the term for the "energetic body," *pranamaya kosha*. Your *prana* stands ready to serve your life and fuel your wellness each time you connect with it.

A Deeper Exploration: The Layers of Your Being (*Koshas*)

Exactly how many bodies can one person have? Yoga philosophy proposes that we each inhabit five distinct "bodies" called **koshas**. These layers of our existence can be thought of using the Sanskrit translation of "sheaths" because, onion-like, they cover our deepest, most essential aspects. The five **koshas**, in other words, surround the ultimate Self that defines each of us:[2]

1. Physical body (matter); *annamaya kosha*
2. Energetic body (life force); *pranamaya kosha*
3. Thought body (mind); *manomaya kosha*
4. Intellectual body (knowledge, awareness, wisdom); *vijnanamaya kosha*
5. Spiritual body (bliss, joy); *anandamaya kosha*

HOW YOGA PHILOSOPHY HELPS US UNDERSTAND ENERGY

When your *prana*, your vital energy, is compromised, you may struggle to feel motivated to actively participate in your life. In the midst of a depressive episode, you may curl up in bed and wonder how you will ever find the energy to rise. You'll question your ability to get up and out the door, to do all the tasks of the day, and to be friendly and kind toward others when you feel terrible about yourself and unable to cope. Thoughts turn dark, and the mind ruminates into hopelessness. Yoga philosophy calls this state an excess of *tamas*, as it is marked by qualities of darkness, inactivity, and lethargy. These states may also manifest as feelings of dullness or melancholia.[3] Perhaps you've used some of those words in describing yourself when you're depressed.

Although the qualities associated with *tamas* are generally considered to be unfavorable and yoga practices aim to reduce its influence, it helps to think about its more positive aspect—that it can supply a "steadying influence in life."[4] We need some amount of *tamas* in our bodies; otherwise we would never rest. But too much darkness and lethargy blocks our ability to be alive in the world.

Rajas describes the qualities of lightness, passion, and action, the opposite of *tamas*. It's important to note that we embody both states at all times, even during depressive episodes. We need a healthy amount of *rajas*—it's what helps us to take action and get things done. But too much *rajas* can lead to an overactive mind, racing thoughts, and feelings of instability and irritability. In the presence of anxiety, yoga practices aim to reduce the influence of *rajas*.

In the midst of some types of depression, your *rajas* is present, but it's—quite literally—depressed. It's not awakened enough to counterbalance the heaviness of your excessive *tamas*. In that case, your goal in yoga practice is to open your physical body and activate your vital energy to decrease *tamas* and increase life force, or *prana*.

In other types of depression, such as agitated depression, the main symptoms of a depressive mood with marked anxiety and restlessness reflect that both *rajas* and *tamas* are in heightened states of activity.[5] In those cases, a yoga practice would be geared toward reducing both *tamas* and *rajas*.

You may recall that there is a third quality of being—*sattva*, meaning balance and harmony. Remember, you carry all three aspects of your being within you at the same time. Through yoga practice, you can adjust the prevalence of *tamas* or *rajas*—or both—and ultimately bring your mind into this peacefully energized state of *sattva*.

YOGA WON'T CHANGE YOU— YOU'LL CHANGE YOURSELF

Part of the elegant beauty of yoga is that it can affect the mind by working with the physical side of your being—your body and your breath. That idea can be freeing when the emotional issues that weigh you down feel overly complex and hard to process. In my view, you don't have to analyze yourself during yoga practice, nor do you need to recount all the experiences in your life that have shaped your moods. Simply paying attention to your body can bring you to a point at which you feel a palpable shift in your emotions. When your energy is low because of depressive symptoms and feelings, this can feel very reassuring. When you focus on your physical experience in your yoga practice, you may actually experience a life-changing shift from inactivity to wanting to be a part of the world, from not caring about yourself or others to feelings of love and passion, a shift from darkness into lightness.

Steve, a participant in our study, exemplified this phenomenon of an emotional energy shift's connections with physical behaviors. Steve was an older man who wasn't used to physical activity because of debilitating back pain. When I met him, I noticed he was slightly hunched over. His shoulders rolled forward, and his chest was a little sunken. It was hard for him to take a full, deep breath. When he talked, he often looked down rather than meeting my eyes, and sometimes he didn't finish his thoughts. As I got to know him, I recognized that his posture wasn't caused by his back pain—it was a physical manifestation of his depression.

Because of his back condition, Steve practiced standing poses with his back against a wall for support. Other poses were also modified so he could experience them comfortably. During the first few weeks of class, he reported muscle soreness, which was not unexpected, but also fatigue and tiredness during and after his sessions. This was the depression talking—it had taken away the vital energy he needed to make it through his day.

As the sessions progressed, yoga started to help his back, and he became aware of his posture. He learned how to stand up tall, with his shoulders back and his chest broad and open, and he was able to breathe more fully. He had more room in his body for breath, and before too long, this translated into having more room in his life for vital energy.

At the end of one class, Steve reported that his mood had noticeably shifted during the session, although he couldn't put his finger on how or why it had happened. This was a turning point for him—I watched him wake up before my eyes, becoming enthusiastic about his yoga practice and interested in how each movement felt. He began verbalizing his thoughts about the poses and reflecting on mood changes he noticed during our classes. He was coming back into his own life—first by fully inhabiting his body, and then by allowing his physical sensations to inform his emotional reality. He was beginning to awaken *rajas* and reduce *tamas* in his system, building a store of the energy he needed to counterbalance his depression and lethargy.

After our time together, Steve wrote a note thanking the study team for helping him change his mood. But the reality was that it was he who had made that change, not the team. By opening himself—literally—to yoga practice, he had become embodied and mentally present, able to understand his experiences on a deeper energetic level. His *tamas* and *rajas* were at more optimal levels, and his mind had found a place of peace.

THREE QUESTIONS TO PREPARE YOU FOR PRACTICE

Before you begin your practice, check in with yourself on these three questions. Do not judge or evaluate your answers. Simply carry them with you through your practice.

1. On a scale of 1 to 10, how would you rate your current energy level?
2. What is one thing in your life that consistently gives you an energy boost?
3. If you had a "full tank" of energy, what would you do?

After your practice, you will have a chance to note any changes in your thoughts and feelings. I chose these poses because they work to open your chest and lift your spine and heart to help you cultivate the qualities of *rajas*—lightness, action, and passion—and integrate those qualities into your daily life. Focus your mind on the sensations that arise as you gently move and open your body, especially in your chest and heart. Perhaps you will notice a swell of vital essential energy. You may find you are carrying yourself with more ease and with your head held high, with dignity. Your breath may flow more smoothly and deeply, and you may find your moods shifting, becoming more harmonious. Be a detective, looking inside yourself for the presence of vital energy that can enliven and support you throughout your day.

YOGA PRACTICE FOR ENERGY

I. Cross-Legged Seated Pose with Ocean Breath

Sit comfortably with your legs crossed on the floor or on a folded blanket, or sit in a chair if that's easier for you. Your spine should be tall and your chest broad and open. Bring your hands together in Prayer Position, palms joined at heart center. Feel the warm energy that is created with your palms together, and let that warmth spread through your arms and into your chest. Create an intention for your practice—to let your body open and receive vital energy. Release your hands and rest them on your thighs in the Gesture of Consciousness.

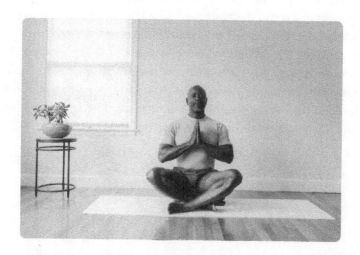

Roll your shoulders back and draw your shoulder blades down from your ears. Bring your ears in line with your shoulders, keeping your chin parallel to the floor. Does this feel different from how you usually sit? You are now sitting with your spine, chest, and head aligned with each other—organized in a way that helps your physical body support itself without straining your muscles. Notice the effect of sitting with your body in alignment. Are your thoughts and feelings quieter? Notice your breath. What is the quality of your inhalations and exhalations? With your chest long and open, perhaps each inhale is longer than usual. Because inhaling activates your body, your inhalation is associated with *rajas*. Let your inhalation deepen and feel breath rising up and awakening your whole being with fresh, vital energy.

Now practice Ocean Breath for two to three minutes, focusing on the fresh, rejuvenating, stimulating energy that each inhalation brings. Begin with a normal inhale, then gently contract your throat muscles and exhale in Ocean Breath. If you are able, inhale in Ocean Breath as well. If that brings on feelings of stress or challenge, try practicing Ocean Breath exhalations only.

2. Hero's Pose with Cow-Face Arms

Sit with your hips on your heels or, if that's not comfortable for you, place a block between your feet and sit on the block. Lift your left arm up, bend your elbow, and take your left hand to the nape of your neck. Hold your left elbow with your right hand, and stretch the left arm upward to open your armpit and shoulder. Now take your right arm down and swing it behind your back. Walk your right hand up your back, reaching your left hand down to meet it, and clasp your fingers. If your hands can't reach each other, drape a belt over your left shoulder and hold it with both hands, letting it make the connection between left and right.

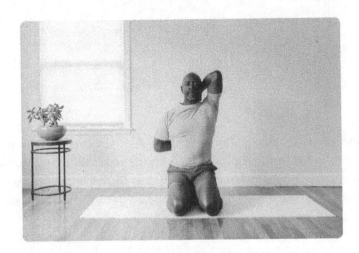

Inhale into the left side of your chest, all the way from your ribs up to your elbow. Reach upward with your left arm as much as possible, noticing your chest and shoulder opening and releasing tension. Hold this stretch for three or four breaths before gently releasing both arms. Repeat on the opposite side. After you've practiced both sides, rest your hands on your thighs, close your eyes, and notice the feeling that you've stretched your chest, shoulders, and upper back. Notice that you're sitting tall, with your chest open and your head high.

3. Energizing Sun Salutation

Stand in Mountain Pose. Close or lower your eyes and meditate for a moment on the qualities of lightness, action, and passion. Imagine how you might feel when you can actually embody those qualities in a consistent, sustainable way. As you practice two rounds of Sun Salutation, feel it bringing your whole body into action and movement. Use your inhalations to invigorate every part of your body, and use your exhales to soften hard places and release tension. As you guide your body into each pose with your breath, can you find lightness, especially in your chest and shoulders? Finally, as your inhalations open your chest, visualize the passion that exists in your heart. Remember, even when you can't feel passion, it is still present within you—it just needs to be awakened and brought into the light. When you are finished with Sun Salutation, stay in Mountain Pose for a few breaths and notice any changes in your physical and mental bodies.

See pages 172–173 for a photographic Sun Salutation refresher.
Mountain Pose
Upward Hand Pose
Standing Forward Bend Pose
Standing Forward Bend Pose—Head Up
Standing Forward Bend Pose
Downward Facing Dog Pose
High Plank Pose
Four Limb Staff Pose
Cobra Pose or Upward Facing Dog Pose
Downward Facing Dog Pose

Standing Forward Bend Pose
Standing Forward Bend Pose—Head Up
Standing Forward Bend Pose
Upward Hand Pose
Mountain Pose

4. Warrior II

Stand with your feet about four feet apart. Turn your left foot in slightly, and turn your right foot and leg out 90 degrees. Stretch your arms apart at shoulder height. Draw your shoulder blades down and away from your ears, noticing how that action helps support and open your chest.

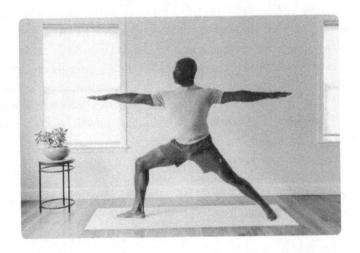

To get ready, press your feet strongly down into the earth and inhale up through your whole body. Start at your feet, breathe up into your legs and then into your trunk, and finally send the flow of breath down the length of your arms. Visualize vitality flowing upward from the earth and throughout your whole body. Stay here for another breath, noticing broadness across your hips, your abdomen, and especially your chest. Can you begin to feel an opening there, space for passion to build in your heart?

On an exhalation, bend your right knee until it is directly over your ankle. Stay in Warrior II for a few breaths, bringing even more vitality into your body as you inhale, and releasing any tension in your shoulders as you exhale. Do you feel the space within broadening and opening even further?

To come out of the pose, straighten your right leg as you inhale. Practice the pose on the opposite side of your body, and then come back to Mountain Pose. Close or lower your eyes and notice openness and lightness in your chest, fresh, vibrant energy flowing through your body, and whispers of passion stirring in your heart.

5. Bridge Pose

Lie down on your back with your knees bent and your feet flat on the floor, about hip distance apart. Draw your tailbone toward your heels, elongating your lower back, and firm your legs and buttocks. Inhaling, slowly lift your hips and trunk upward while your shoulders and head remain on the floor. Lift your hips only as far as you can while keeping your lower back long and comfortable.

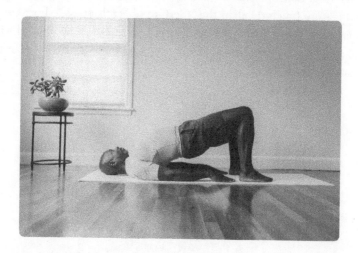

Hold the pose for a few breaths while you feel how your spine lifts, bringing lightness and space into your chest. Notice how your breath seems to fill your chest and linger there. You may want to stay in the pose for a few extra moments, just enjoying the reservoir of vital energy and stamina that you are building. While exhaling, slowly release the pose vertebra by vertebra, starting from your upper spine and laying your spine down on the floor as you visualize vital energy and fortitude flowing fully through your body. Repeat Bridge Pose two more times, visualizing your reservoir of *prana* awakening your whole being each time. After you've finished, draw your knees into your chest and hug them, releasing any tension in your lower back.

6. Marichi's Twist I

Sit with your legs straight, your spine tall, and your chest broad and open. Sit on a blanket if your hips tip back. Bend your right knee and place your foot on the floor. Take your left hand behind you to the floor, and reach upward with your right arm. Stay here for a couple of breaths, leaning back a bit to lift your trunk upward, and notice the newly discovered reservoir of energy rising up through your body. Keeping your chest open, turn your trunk to the left and place your right arm inside your right leg. Bend your elbow and open your palm, bringing your right hand into a hand gesture (*mudra*) called the "Gesture of Fearlessness."[6] Imagine yourself as being fearless in your journey into well-being. Lift your spine upward with each inhale, and deepen your twist as you exhale. Turning the right side of your trunk to

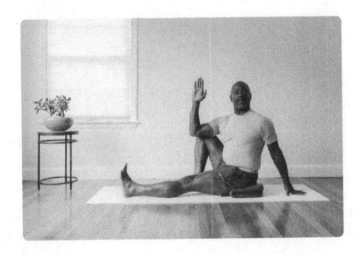

the left, visualize your chest turning toward a vibrant and energizing light. To come out of the pose, inhale and lift your arms up while you turn your trunk back to center. Change legs, and practice the pose on the opposite side.

7. Seated Forward Bend Pose

Sit with your legs extended in front of you. Adjust your trunk so it is upright. If your hips tip backward, sit on a folded blanket. For more support, sit on two side-by-side blocks (pictured). Lift your arms upward as you inhale, and exhaling, fold forward from your hip joints and bring your hands to your feet. Hold your feet with a belt or bend your knees if you can't easily reach your feet or if your back feels any discomfort. Keeping your eyes open and your gaze soft, notice the sensations in the back of your body. Can you feel a comfortable, sustainable stretch along your legs, hips, and spine? Seated Forward Bend really works your hamstrings, the muscles in the backs of your thighs, so channel the inner fearlessness you cultivated in Marichi's Twist I and breathe deeply, keeping your mind present to each moment and the sensations that arise. As you inhale, visualize tight muscles becoming long and soft, and then let the tension within them go as you exhale.

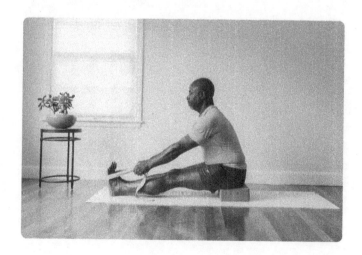

When you're ready to come out of the pose, lift your arms and trunk upward as you inhale, reaching your arms up over your head. Then release your hands to your sides as you exhale. Sit for a few moments and notice if your body is a little quieter and your thoughts are a bit lighter.

8. Energizing Inverted Pose

Sit with one hip against a wall, lie down, and swing your legs up the wall. Slide a bolster under your hips to come into Inverted Pose. Once your body is comfortable, focus your mind on your chest. Notice how energy flows from your legs to your hips, pooling briefly in your hips before flowing into your chest. With your hips and lower back in this lifted position and your neck long on the floor, your chin and chest move gently toward one another. In yoga philosophy, this position encourages the energy, or *prana*, that has flowed into your chest to be held there as it freely bathes your lungs and heart. Your heart center can now become a reservoir of vitality, an infinite wellspring of energy, stamina, and inner strength.

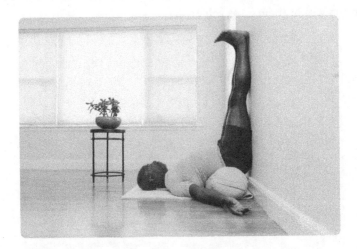

9. Deep Relaxation with Ocean Breath—
Your Awakened, Energized Self

Lie down with a folded blanket under your head and a bolster under your knees. Be sure your shoulders, arms, and feet rest evenly on the earth.

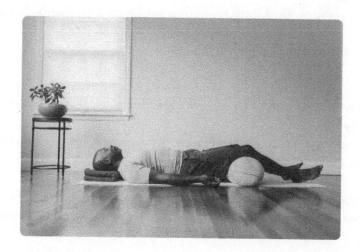

Lower your eyelids or close your eyes. Breathe smoothly and evenly in and out, visualizing your breath rising gently up from the base of your spine into your chest and releasing from your chest all the way down to your feet. As you rest with your body in stillness, visualize the energy you have found during this practice, the life force that flows through the energetic layer of your body as a life-supporting, vibrating, shimmering current that moves through your whole being.

During your practice you've awakened *rajas*, the energy of action and passion. Now those qualities are alive within you and available for you to use to help get out of bed in the morning and sustain yourself throughout your day—each and every day. As you rest in Deep Relaxation, let it be with the comforting understanding that you can build up your energy whenever you feel fatigued and lethargic from depression. You are never devoid of *rajas*, even in a state of deep depression. It is always part of your essence; now you have new ways to access and activate this energizing force. After you have rested in Deep Relaxation for a few minutes, practice five to six rounds of Ocean Breath, and feel energy flowing through your body.

When you are ready, release your Ocean Breath and take a couple of normal breaths. Transition into your twenty-minute Coherent Breathing practice, using your timer or app to track your smooth, even breaths (six-second inhales and six-second exhales are a good goal).

When you've finished, turn your attention back to the questions you asked yourself before your practice. How has your experience affected your understanding of how energy works in your body and mind?

1. On a scale of 1 to 10, how would you rate your current energy level?
2. What was one thing you experienced in the practice that gave you an energy boost?
3. Is there an energizing lesson you can take from your practice into the rest of your day?

Keep your mental focus on the vibrating, sparkling, ever-present reservoir of energy in your body, and the vitality that now supports your journey into well-being.

CHAPTER 8

CALM

Quiet your mind and notice the peace
that's already within you.

A nxiety lives in a too-fast world. In anxiety, breath, movement, and thoughts all race, leaving us breathlessly dreaming of what it might be like to move through each day in a state of calm. In this yearned-for calmness, our frenetic actions would slow, our minds would be present and focused, and we would experience physical as well as mental release from fear and worry. This peaceful existence sounds wonderful—but anxiety can make it feel like a horizon that slips away each time we draw closer to it. We may be able to find moments of calm during our day, but with anxiety thrumming in our ears, abiding inner peace feels nearly unattainable.

You're not alone if you struggle to find physical and emotional calm on a regular basis. The comedian and television host Ellen DeGeneres put it well when she quipped, "I get these fleeting, beautiful moments of inner peace and stillness, and then the other twenty-three hours and forty-five minutes of the day, I'm a human trying to make it through in this world."[1]

Getting calm and staying calm isn't easy for anyone, whether or not they suffer from clinical anxiety. After all, the world we live in *is* fast, maybe even too fast.

WHAT IS CALM?

Dictionary definitions of calm often have to do with the absence of something—strong emotions like anger or nervousness, violent weather like wind, or confrontational actions like raised voices. In this way, calm is understood as a kind of stillness.

But calm is not the absence of all action. It's not frozen or stagnant; it's intentional and present. It's worth reflecting on the fact that "calm" is also a verb. To calm someone or something is to bring it into a state of tranquility, to soothe or quiet a frenetic feeling, person, or space. This process of calming is peaceful, but active. Yoga philosophy embraces both these definitions, offering that calm is both a state of being and an action that is within our power to take.

In yoga, it is accepted as a premise that a deep sense of calm exists within each of us. So too do pure joy and happiness. These qualities are considered to be the very essence of our inner nature, the "birthright" we discussed in Chapter 2. In the throes of anxiety, when your thoughts are overwhelming and you feel stuck ruminating about the past or worrying about the future, it may be impossible to believe that you can ever find happiness, let alone a sense of peace. But if you accept that peace and calm are innate in your nature, you can begin to turn inward and look for where they abide. This may seem like an enormous task, but be assured that a calm, quiet place already exists within you, and with the simple techniques you will learn in this chapter to slow down your breath, movements, and thoughts, you will be able to find that place.

A Deeper Exploration: Inner Peace (Shanti)

The Sanskrit word for peace and tranquility is **shanti**. Other definitions include rest, calmness, and bliss. It is the concept of **shanti** that I'm referring to when I say that yoga philosophy accepts as a premise that peace and joy reside in each of us—the meanings of **shanti** also reflect the way in which yoga philosophy connects calmness with happiness. Many yoga talks or meditations are concluded when the yogi or yogini says, "Om shanti, shanti, shanti," which is meant as an invocation of peace upon all who listened to the teaching. The same phrase is often shared at the end of a yoga class, or chanted as a personal mantra. Uttering **shanti** three times is believed to bestow peace on the mind, body, and spirit—the three principal parts of our existence.[2]

HOW YOGA CREATES CALM TO EASE ANXIETY

You have learned about some of the characteristics of depression in yogic terms—inertia, inactivity, and darkness (*tamas* in Sanskrit). You have also learned about the qualities of *rajas*—action, passion, restlessness, and irritability. According to yoga philosophy, we have (and need) both *tamas* and *rajas* within us at all times. And we know from Western science that depression and anxiety often coexist in individuals. According to yoga philosophy, if our *tamas* is excessive, depressive symptoms may dominate. The reverse is true in anxiety and in other nervous system conditions such as post-traumatic stress disorder. In these anxious states, a disproportionate level of *rajas* leads to an overactive mind that is drawn all too quickly from one concern to the next, more quickly than it can process each thought. When both depression and anxiety disorders are found in the same person, such as someone who has Major Depressive Disorder and PTSD, *tamas* and *rajas* may both be excessive relative to the needs of the moment. In all of these cases, a balanced practice of yoga postures and breath work can reduce heightened *tamas* and/or *rajas*, and will help to cultivate a state of calm harmony, or *sattva*.

Let's review how anxiety works biologically—then you will see how directly yoga calms bodies and minds. When you feel anxious, your nervous system might be overly sensitive to external stimuli. Your vagus nerve sends messages to alert your brain to a potentially stressful or even dangerous situation. In response to this perception of danger, accurate or inaccurate, your body responds with increased mental activity. This activates the fight-or-flight response of your autonomic nervous system. Stress hormones are released and your heart rate and breath rate increase, all in an effort to meet the challenges—real or imagined—that your mind thinks are in front of you. This is not an inherently negative process—stress hormones and increased heart rate and breathing help us respond to challenges. But in a chronic "stress cycle," your entire system can remain frenzied for too long, spinning like wheels on a car that's not in gear.

Yoga can help address the ways stress and anxiety tax your physical and emotional bodies. William J. Broad, the author of *The Science of Yoga: The Risks and the Rewards*, concluded, "If yoga does one thing, it relaxes you."[3]

Sometimes during and usually after a yoga practice, your heart rate slows and your breath becomes more relaxed. Your resilience, the ability to encounter challenges and rebound from them, increases. In those moments, you are experiencing the deactivation of the fight-or-flight response, the critical ability of your body to return to a state of relaxed alertness.[4] Without the ability to return to calmness, your body would remain in a heightened response state, which could lead to additional physical and mental maladies. Depression, PTSD, and chronic pain are all known to be conditions that are exacerbated by stress.[5]

By asking your body to move in new ways, yoga poses provide opportunities to experience healthy stress, and then to practice transitioning from agitation into calmness. When we learn new types of movements, we get to explore our discomfort and then recover.

Stephanie, who participated in our study, experienced this type of resilience when she practiced a standing backbend that was challenging for her. The first step of the pose involved raising her arms over her head and touching a wall close behind her. She got her fingers to the wall just fine, but then worriedly said, "I can't breathe!" Her breath had instantly become quick and shallow—I immediately recognized it as an anxious breath.

The physical action of the pose may have been her trigger—she said she felt ungrounded and insecure trying to hold the backbend for even a few moments. She tried again and had the same experience with her breath, only this time her body started to shake as well. She came out of the pose and took a rest.

I suggested that instead of trying to breathe comfortably while holding the pose, she could try practicing it with constant movement—a slow inhalation to bring her arms up and back to the wall, and a deep, long exhalation while bringing her arms right back down. She did this with ease, and the look on her face transformed from worried to tranquil. She was able to control her breath so that she could inhale and exhale fully, and the calm smile on her face as she finished showed that by working with her body and breath, she had changed her state of mind. Shifting her approach from a sustained, held pose to one of constant movement helped her meet her overactive mind where it was, so her mind could gradually slow down over the course of a few cycles moving in and out of the pose.

THE CALMING POWER OF THE BREATH

You are probably used to hearing a friend or family member say "Just take a deep breath" when you're feeling anxious or upset. Maybe you even murmur that instruction to yourself when you're in a heightened state of worry or stress. They are wise words—the way we breathe directly affects our ability to feel physical and emotional calm.

The two halves of each breath—inhaling and exhaling—create opposite responses in your body: each breath in activates the sympathetic nervous system, while each breath out is associated with parasympathetic nervous system activity. We can use this to our advantage when we leverage our breathing for emotional well-being. As you've been learning in each practice chapter, you can take deep inhalations when you need to build energy, and you should deepen your exhalations to slow your heart rate and quiet your mind. The shift from an overactive mind to a calm one can be experienced in just a few minutes when the focus on breath shifts to exhalation. It can feel astonishing the first time you experience it.

Try this simple breathing exercise to feel this calming effect. Sit comfortably in a chair with your feet on the floor, or lie down with your head resting on a folded blanket. Lower your eyelids or close your eyes. Breathe into your belly, and let your exhalation come out slowly, so that it's longer than your inhalation. Repeat this for five or six breaths. Notice the sensations in your abdomen and your chest as you inhale, and notice how they change as you exhale.

When you are done, notice your body and your thoughts, and then gently open your eyes. Perhaps you let go of a little tension in your belly, and maybe there is space in your mind for your thoughts to exist without colliding. Perhaps you are able to feel less judgmental of yourself, and a little kinder toward others.

THE PATH TO A CALMER LIFE STARTS
WITH KNOWING YOURSELF

I've been using the word "notice" throughout this book—have you, ahem, noticed? This is very deliberate, to remind you that self-reflection is at the core of yoga practice. As the yoga master B. K. S. Iyengar put it, "You cannot hope to experience inner peace or freedom without understanding the workings of your mind."[6]

When you take time to practice yoga, you give yourself the gift of quiet space—time to yourself—in which you can reflect on your thoughts and emotions. As you recognize your behavior patterns, you gain insight into your past and how it affects your actions in the present. As you work with your anxiety, you learn to understand and accept yourself through movement and breath practices. This is a powerful skill that you can use to calm yourself in any given moment and, ultimately, to transform your emotional life.

We might think the best way to manage anxiety is to put words to our fears; we've discussed before how powerful it is to name a feeling or emotion. And it's true—writing in a journal or talking to a therapist or trusted friend is certainly part of the healing path. However, when we practice yoga, we come to understand that talking alone may not be enough to convince the brain to calm its signal patterns. We also need to move and breathe in a way that lets our bodies and minds rest, quiet, and calm down. Noticing yourself, mindfully understanding and recognizing yourself, is a key part of this process.

Bessel van der Kolk, the psychiatrist and trauma expert, says "embodied" practices like yoga cultivate lasting physical and emotional calm because they nurture mindful habits. Teaching people to achieve focused presence in the here and now is, in van der Kolk's view, "the great challenge" of helping traumatized people heal.[7] The same could be said for anxiety that is not related to trauma. In yoga, you learn to fully and deeply notice yourself—your body, your mind, and your emotions.

Paying attention to yourself will start to help as soon as you use it to understand your physiological condition, noticing whether your heart is racing or beating at a resting rate, whether your breaths are long and smooth or short and shallow. Paying attention to the sensations in your physical body gives you crucial information about the state of your mind. Your breaths and heart rate can be thought of as indicators of your mood; the speed of those physical activities reflects the pace of your thoughts.

The more comfortable you get mindfully noticing these signals, the more you will learn to trust yourself. Instead of being pushed and pulled in all directions by your emotions, you will find that you can slow down, take some deep breaths, and find stable ground on which to stand. Whether there is a tornado of thoughts swirling around in your head, or whether you feel "shut down" and can't think at all, you can find a strong, calm center within, an oasis of calm, simply by bringing your attention to your breath, simply by listening to your heart.

Yet there may be times when your anxiety is stronger than your breath—when you can't breathe deeply, or when you can't slow your breath rate down enough to lengthen your exhales. Think back on Stephanie's experience in the standing backbend. She needed support to learn how to pay mindful attention to her body's stress signals. In short order, she was able to redirect her movements so that her physical and emotional systems could regulate. See if you can approach your practice with the same openness, if you can listen to what your body is telling you it needs to find calm.

THREE QUESTIONS TO PREPARE YOU FOR PRACTICE

Before you begin, ask yourself these three questions. Notice your responses to each, but do not judge or wrestle with them. There is a special emphasis in this calming practice on meeting your body and mind wherever they are. Embrace your starting place as you check in with yourself.

1. How would you describe your breath pattern and heart rate right now?
2. What does anxiety feel like in your body? What does calm feel like?
3. Can you think of a place, a person, or an object that you consistently associate with calmness?

After your practice, you will have a chance to check in with yourself again to see if your perspective has changed, if your thinking has clarified, or if any anxiety has lifted. This practice should help address anxiety because it offers a level of movement that aligns with the level of energy you are experiencing. Since anxiety produces a lot of energy—excessive energy, in fact—we'll meet your mind where it is. When your body is a little calmer, you'll slow your movements and thoughts with poses that draw you inward, so you can let go of the world around you, learn about yourself, and find a place of trust within. Your Deep Relaxation will bring you back to the premise we discussed at the beginning of this chapter—that happiness and joy, peace and calm are parts of your inner nature, so much so that you can keep yourself relaxed, serene, and peaceful, even in the presence of anxiety and stress.

YOGA PRACTICE FOR CALM

I. Cross-Legged Seated Pose with Ocean Breath

Sit comfortably with your legs crossed on the floor or on a folded blanket, or sit in a chair if its comfort beckons. Your spine should lift up and your chest should be broad and open. Lower your eyelids or close your eyes and bring your hands together at your heart center, in Prayer Position. Create an intention in this pose—let yourself know that you will take time to notice your thoughts and the sensations in your body. If you recall this intention often, you will learn which thoughts are trying to hijack your mind, and which thoughts can help you understand your deepest feelings and increase your self-confidence. In this way, you will create a basis of self-trust that can help you feel grounded whenever your emotions try to pull you into a tailspin. After a few breaths, once you feel settled in your intention, release your hands and rest them on your thighs in the Gesture of Consciousness.

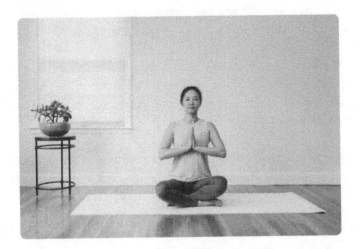

For this calming practice, you will focus on Ocean Breath exhalations. Take a normal inhale, pause at the top, and gently contract your throat muscles to create an Ocean Breath as you breathe out. Feel how Ocean Breath gently elongates your exhalations. Do not worry about how long each breath actually is. Just enjoy the feeling of letting go of stress and becoming grounded in your intention with each elongated Ocean Breath exhale. Practice for two to three minutes, knowing you can release Ocean Breath at any time if you start to feel anxious or confused. After you have finished, sit quietly, feel your body rooted to the earth, and experience how that grounding begins to tamp down the rapid pace of your thoughts.

2. Reclining Hand-to-Big-Toe Poses I and II

Lie on your back with a belt by your side. Support your head on a folded blanket if that is comfortable. Take a few moments to feel that your body is well-grounded, and observe how your mind can relax when you are physically supported. Perhaps your thoughts can become a little calmer. Draw your right knee into your chest and place your belt around the ball of your foot. Inhale and stretch your right leg up toward the sky while you keep your left leg grounded. Hold your belt with your right hand. If this strains your hips or back, you can bend your left knee as much as you need to feel comfortable. Use the flow of your breath to create gentle movements in your lifted right leg—as you inhale, stretch up through your leg, and as you exhale, draw your foot toward your head by any amount possible. Notice how the sensations in your legs change as your breath shifts.

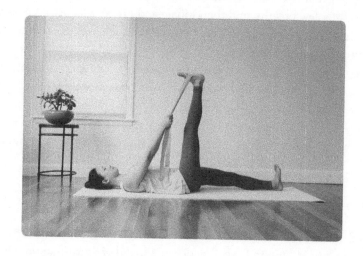

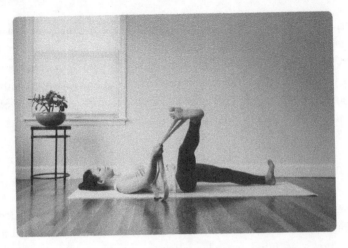

After a few breaths, extend your left arm straight out from your shoulder, and draw your right leg down to the right as you exhale. Notice new sensations that come into your right leg—where does the stretch go now? Take your leg down toward the floor only as much as allows you to feel a comfortable, sustainable stretch along your inner right leg. You should not feel strain, especially on the inside of your knee. For less stretch, rest your right foot on a support—a block or bolster if your foot is near the floor, or a chair if your foot is higher up. Keep both sides of your trunk long and your chest broad, and be sure your shoulders are relaxed. Remain in this stretch for a few breaths, and then inhale and lift your leg back up toward the sky before releasing your belt and bringing your right leg back onto your mat. Rest for a few breaths, and repeat the pose on your opposite side.

The movements in this pose stretch the backs of your legs, your hips, and your lower back, releasing tension and promoting lower body flexibility. As you practice, keep your hips and trunk evenly grounded. Notice that by grounding some parts of your body, you can find a feeling of freedom—perhaps a sense of calmness—somewhere else within yourself, whether it is in your legs, your hips, or your mind.

3. Calming Sun Salutation

Now you will meet your active mind and body with active movement. Stand at the top of your mat in Mountain Pose. Practice one round of Sun Salutation, breathing in and out evenly. Move at a comfortable pace, feeling your body actively transitioning from one pose to the next. Follow your breath, and notice that the sensations in your body may change with each movement. For your second round, practice with your mind focused on the length of your exhalations. Can they be long and complete? Can you feel how a different approach to exhaling starts to change your thoughts?

See pages 172–173 for a photographic Sun Salutation refresher.
Mountain Pose
Upward Hand Pose
Standing Forward Bend Pose
Standing Forward Bend Pose—Head Up
Standing Forward Bend Pose
Downward Facing Dog Pose
High Plank Pose
Four Limb Staff Pose
Cobra Pose or Upward Facing Dog Pose
Downward Facing Dog Pose
Standing Forward Bend Pose
Standing Forward Bend Pose—Head Up
Standing Forward Bend Pose
Upward Hand Pose
Mountain Pose

4. Wide-Legged Standing Forward Bend Pose

Stand with your feet four to five feet apart, with your toes facing straight forward. Place your hands on your hips and fold forward from your hip joints. Place your hands on the floor or on a pair of blocks. While inhaling, lift your trunk halfway up and look forward, and as you exhale, release your trunk toward the floor. If this is difficult, bend your knees.

With your feet grounded and your legs strong and stable, focus on your breath. With each inhale breathe up from the earth into your legs, and with each long, deep, full exhale, release your hips, trunk, heart, and head toward the earth. If you are comfortable, you can close your eyes partly or entirely. Feel your eyes turning

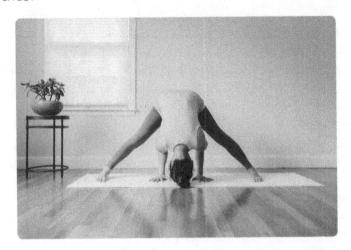

away from the outside world; imagine you could look within yourself. Notice your changing thoughts, wherever they are in this moment, and then visualize a place of stability within yourself, a place that doesn't change when your emotions do. Stay in the pose for a few breaths and rest in a feeling of support and steadiness. Place your hands on your hips and lift your trunk upward as you inhale. Bring your feet together and stand in Mountain Pose for a few breaths.

5. Standing Backbend Pose

You'll practice this pose just as Stephanie did—in a slow flow, moving in and out of the pose to the rhythm of your breath, once again using movement and breath to meet your mind where it is. Stand in Mountain Pose with your back just a few inches from a wall. Inhale slowly and lift your arms up, coming into Upward Hand Pose. With your knees slightly bent and your chest lifted, reach backward and touch your hands to the wall. Exhale slowly while bringing your arms away from the wall and down to your sides. Repeat this flow two more times, mindfully noticing that your breath and movements reflect the level of energy you feel in your body. Experience your breath and the movements of your body acting in sync with each other in a rhythmic, inte-grated connection of body and mind. When you are finished, take a moment to stand in Mountain Pose with your eyes closed or lowered. Notice any difference in your thoughts. Perhaps there are fewer of them, and perhaps they are quieter.

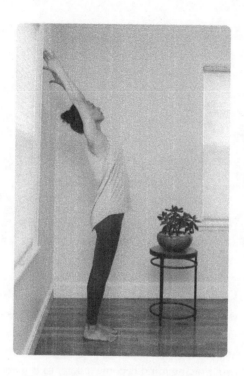

6. Reclining Bound Angle Pose

Have a stack of three or four blankets or a bolster within reach. Either place your bolster lengthwise on your mat or fold two blankets, stack them, and place them in the same position. Fold another blanket and place it across the top of your bolster or stack of blankets to form a T-shape. Sit in front of the props, with your hips about four inches in front of the bottom of the bolster or lengthwise blankets. Lie down with your trunk supported on the bolster or long blankets and your head on the horizontal blanket. Bend your knees and bring the soles of your feet together, relaxing your knees out to the sides. You might like to place blocks under your thighs to ensure your inner thighs are very comfortable. For extra relaxation, place a folded blanket across your abdomen.

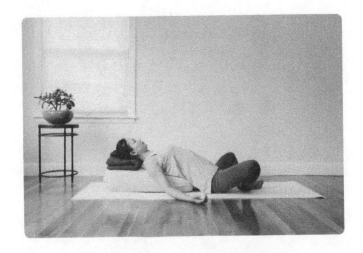

Lower your eyelids or close your eyes. Inhale softly up from the base of your spine all the way to the crown of your head. Let your exhale become long and follow it as it flows gently from the crown of your head to the base of your spine. Feel your chest soft and expansive, the outer layers of your body releasing. Notice that your energy level is calming down. Feel your racing mind become quieter as it is able to focus inward.

Remain in the pose for five minutes. To come out, use your hands to help your thighs come together, and roll onto one side. Come up to a seated position.

7. Child's Pose

Sit with your knees bent, resting your hips on or between your feet, depending on your comfort level. If your hips do not reach your feet, place a folded blanket, block, or bolster between your legs for more support. Inhale and reach your arms above your head, bringing length into your trunk. As you exhale, bend at your hips and extend your arms and upper body forward. Rest your head on the floor or on a block.

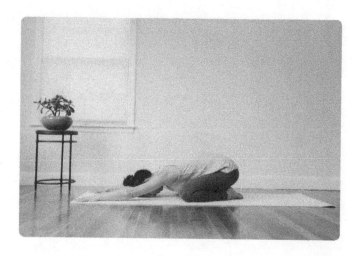

Child's Pose is one of the most calming and restorative poses in yoga. It is a beautifully peaceful way to rest your body between your backbend and the forward bend you will practice next.

8. Seated Forward Bend Pose with Head Supported

Sit with your legs straight out in front of you and your trunk lifted upright. If this is challenging or if your back is uncomfortable, sit on a folded blanket and bend your knees slightly. With an inhalation, raise your arms up to lift your heart, and as you exhale, bend forward from your hips and hold your feet, either with your hands or with a belt. Stay here for a couple of breaths and feel your body adjusting to the pose.

Fold forward to the extent that is comfortable for you, elongating your trunk toward your feet. Support your head by putting blocks on or between your legs—or even resting your forehead on the seat of a chair—meeting your body wherever it is. Do not force yourself to go forward if your body isn't ready. Your body should feel a comfortable and sustainable stretch, and your mind should feel a sense of quiet and relaxation as your gaze softens and your attention softly turns inward. Focus your mind on the changing physical sensations in your body and on the ebb and flow of your thoughts. Notice that challenging or uncomfortable emotions can bubble up

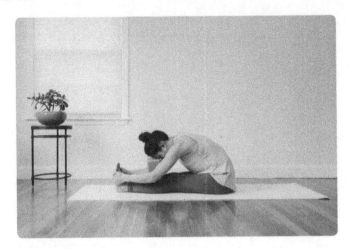

but then drift away. Feel how in this restorative pose, space appears for constructive, supportive thoughts to replace negative ones.

Seated forward bends can be challenging when you first practice them. If you practice this pose consistently, though, you will notice your physical body releasing—especially those pesky hamstring muscles along the backs of your thighs—and your mental body becoming more content. Over time, discomfort can change into comfort and calm, both physically and mentally.

9. Calming Inverted Pose

Sit with your side next to a wall, lie down, and swing your legs up the wall. Slide a bolster under your hips to come into Inverted Pose. Since you've practiced this pose before, you can try experimenting with it by adding a folded blanket on top of the bolster. More height under your hips creates more length along the front of your body, which offers more space for *prana* to flow into your chest as you achieve a deeper inverted position.

Once you are comfortable, lower your eyelids or close your eyes, and return once again to a breathing pattern with a normal inhale and a longer, deeper exhale. Remember, it doesn't matter how much longer your exhalation is. Just let your breath move into an organic rhythm. Each breath in should feel nourishing, and

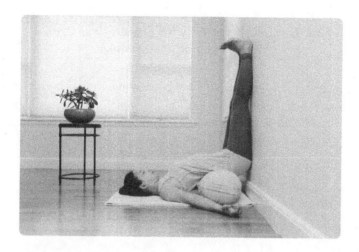

each breath out should deepen your experience and understanding of where you are in this present moment.

Can you notice unhappy, challenging, or ruminating thoughts becoming quieter? When thoughts drift away, there's room for new thoughts to be planted, their seeds sowed and cultivated through your practice of mindful presence. The Buddhist meditation teacher Thich Nhat Hanh is known for saying, "The quality of your life depends on the seeds you water. If you plant tomato seeds in your gardens, tomatoes will grow. Just so, if you water a seed of peace in your mind, peace will grow. When the seeds of happiness in you are watered, you will become happy. When the seed of anger in you is watered, you will become angry. The seeds that are watered frequently are those that will grow strong."[8]

In the beginning of this chapter I introduced the yogic concept that a deep sense of calm, joy, and happiness are all part of your inherent nature—they are the seeds that already live in your heart, even if you have not sensed them recently. In your practice, you have created space for those seeds of peace and joy to take root in your everyday life. Following Thich Nhat Hanh's advice, water your seeds often by acknowledging them as you practice. When you do that mindfully and consistently, you can trust they will come into full bloom.

10. Deep Relaxation with Ocean Breath—
Your Tranquil, Calm Mind

Lie down in a comfortable position. Place a bolster under your knees for more comfort in your lower back. Support your head so that your chin can gently nod toward
your heart, and let your anxious mind bow to the wisdom you have planted and
awakened in yourself.

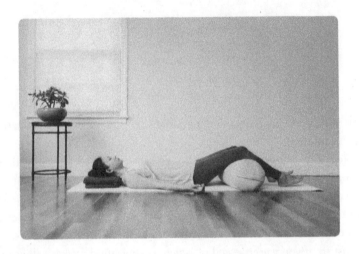

Once you are settled, inhale normally, gently contract your throat muscles, and
exhale and create the sound of an inner sigh. Practice five to six rounds of Ocean
Breath with the awareness that if you practice Ocean Breath inhalations, each one
gently opens the exterior of your body, letting in new, fresh energy. At the same
time, each long, deep Ocean Breath exhalation takes your mind one more step toward calm. In the moments between your breaths, listen for the peace and joy that
always exist within yourself. Perhaps they have a message for you, reminding you
that happiness is your birthright. Or perhaps there is just calmness and stillness, like
a lake's mirrored surface when the wind stops and all of nature becomes quiet. In
either case, find a sense of contentment in which you can rest. Let go of any urge or
desire to act or move. Simply use each breath to take you deeper into calmness and

happiness. Perhaps you are finding these feelings again after a long absence. Give yourself time to re-experience them.

Let yourself be surrounded by contentment until you feel there is nothing pressing or urgent to demand your attention, nothing you need to do or think or feel right now. Just feel the calmness that infuses every part of your body and follow it into your deepest self, where you will find the essential energy in your heart that is *shanti*, the profound and complete peace that is your true nature, your ever-present reservoir of calm, especially in the presence of anxiety and stress.

When you have finished Ocean Breath, take a few normal breaths. Now you are ready to move on to your twenty-minute Coherent Breathing practice, using your timer or app to track breaths that are long and even—aim for six-second inhalations and six-second exhalations. Visualize the quality of *shanti*, of calmness and deep peace, as a gentle energetic shower that flows softly over your body. With each inhale, *shanti* flows into you. With each exhale, let yourself release something—a thought, an emotion, a belief—anything that holds you back from accessing the presence of joy, happiness, and calm in your heart.

When you have finished your practice, take a moment to turn your attention back to the questions you explored at the beginning of this chapter. Notice whether you have a new perspective on your ability to access a place of calm and peace within yourself.

1. What do you notice about your breath pattern and heart rate now?
2. How would you describe any calmness you've discovered during your practice?
3. Was there a particular pose or action in this practice that helped you feel calm?

As you water the seeds of calmness within you, you will surely watch them come into the full bloom of inner peace.

CHAPTER 9

BALANCE

Step back from extremes to come into a place of peaceful harmony.

magine you are a child playing on a swing set. In order to be any fun, the swing has to be moving—forward and backward, up and down. Joyfully, you are propelled skyward, and then you swoop back effortlessly, each moment bringing a new vantage point from which to survey the world around you. Sometimes, you might pump your strong legs a little too hard, causing the swing's chains to buckle and jerk. But quickly you reconnect with the right rhythm for your body, bringing your swing back into its exhilarating equilibrium, coordinating the movements of your legs with the lean of your upper body so you become a human pendulum, collecting the breeze as you breathe between smile-parted lips.

In that moment, see yourself in a blissful state of balance.

There's a reason so many childhood games focus on balance—the seesaw, balance beam, and even a yo-yo come to mind. Through balance-oriented play, children learn how to stay grounded and joyful as they move through the world. They learn to go and return, rise and fall, and then rise again. They learn to stay present at each step along the way, and to trust that they can remain safe and content through all the comings and goings of life.

This quest for balance is the work of a lifetime. As adults, we continue to seek it. The phrase "work-life balance" is common in our culture—we yearn to care for ourselves, our families, and our careers in balanced proportions.

When we struggle emotionally, though, we can feel like we're on a swing that is not under our control. In the inertia of depression, our movement is muted, slow, and devoid of joy. In the frenzy of anxiety, our swing twists and flops in a disorganized, disorienting way. In many, both depressive and anxious symptoms tangle together, coexisting in the same person.

A balanced existence, one that is grounded in clarity and self-awareness, is attainable even in those with a complex set of emotional challenges. Beyond a heavy, depressed mind and an overactive, anxious state is that breezy, sunny pleasure of swinging back and forth in a state of equilibrium. On your journey toward wellness, you are learning to understand your body's and mind's needs in various mood states. The more you develop this self-knowledge, the more accessible a balanced mind-set will feel as you face all of life's complex realities.

It's never too late to reconnect with the joyous equilibrium of a child at play. You are already on the journey toward this self-loving, healthy, emotionally balanced life.

HOW YOGA BRINGS YOU INTO BALANCE

In earlier chapters, we explored the concepts of *rajas*, *tamas*, and *sattva*, qualities that inhabit every object in the universe, including the human body and mind. You may recall that *rajas* is a very active quality, encompassing movement, restlessness, and passion. *Tamas*, by contrast, is lethargic, inactive, and still. For our purposes, we consider excessive *rajas* and *tamas* to roughly correlate with common symptoms of anxiety and depression, respectively.

Imagine a set of scales stacked with equally weighted discs. In the presence of depression, too many weights sit on the *tamas* side of the scale, leaving us low on energy and motivation. Our work, then, is to remove enough discs from the *tamas* side to allow life force to flow freely through the body and mind. In the presence of anxiety, when we feel agitated and unfocused, we find ourselves with too many discs on the *rajas* side of the scales. In that case, we must address the excess by removing enough discs from the *rajas* side to allow for stability. The balance we seek is between action and inaction, between stillness and activity, and between darkness and light. In yoga philosophy, this state of harmony and balance in which *tamas* and *rajas* are at optimal levels is called *sattva*.

A Deeper Exploration:
Action, Inertia, and Balance (Gunas)[1]

Rajas, *tamas*, and *sattva*—activity, lethargy, and harmony—are not independent concepts in yoga philosophy. They are the three **gunas**, or strands, that yoga philosophy suggests make up the entire universe. Each object, each feeling, each person—everything in the whole universe—is made up of these three forces in some relationship to each other. In yoga philosophy, the **gunas** are believed to be permanent, with origins in the primordial world. But each interaction among them is fleeting, passing with time to transition into another ratio of action, rest, and balance. If you are struggling with imbalanced feelings in your day, remember that you have the power to recalibrate, restart, and reimagine the interplay among these three eternal forces at any time.

We practice yoga poses to find physical equilibrium in our bodies, with the expectation that emotional and spiritual balance will follow. In this physical realm, we might even imagine ourselves again like children at play, using our movements to educate ourselves about how we can remain present, safe, and joyful as we modulate between the extremes of life. The yoga teacher and psychologist Bo Forbes explores this idea in her book, *Yoga for Emotional Balance*. She writes of yoga as "a firsthand, embodied experience of our fluctuating emotional landscapes."[2] In other words, if life is a swing, yoga is a tool we can wield to make the ride smoother and more joyful. As we practice, we will become less reactive, more self-aware, and more resilient when challenges arise.

Yoga philosophers have long mined the interplay of physical and mental, spiritual and emotional, all in pursuit of a profound life balance. One of the clearest statements about this comes from Patañjali's *Yoga Sutras*: when we practice yoga postures in a stable, comfortable, and effortless way, we are "no longer upset by the play of opposites."[3] This is one of the most succinct ways to articulate how yoga can bring freedom from the extreme emotions and symptoms we often experience in anxiety and depression. Yoga practice helps us to find a balance amid extreme states, leading us toward a place of peaceful equanimity.

VISUALIZATIONS TO HELP YOU MOVE TOWARD BALANCE

Mood challenges like depression and anxiety and their combinations are, by definition, imbalanced states of being. They tug us away from the balanced center of our emotional scales and toward the outskirts of excessive *rajas* and *tamas*. They affect our thoughts and feelings, as well as our physical postures. You may have even heard your depression or anxiety described as a "chemical imbalance."

In Chapter 5, our centering practice, you worked to bring evenness into your breath, taking a brief pause, a moment of stillness, between inhalations and exhalations. Let's do two similar exercises now, working in the first one with the image of the scales we have been discussing so far in this chapter.

Sit comfortably with your eyes lowered or closed. Without changing your breathing pattern or doing any work at all, identify the emotions that are present for you in this moment. Are you drawn toward a happy emotion or toward a sad, upsetting one? If you notice multiple emotions in your mind at the same time, you are in good company. It's normal to be attracted to happy emotions and to have an aversion to challenging ones, but sometimes the difficult emotions are the "squeaky wheels" that draw our attention. There is nothing wrong with either happy or upsetting emotions, of course; remember that happiness is your birthright, and emotional challenges are part of the human experience. But the swing of emotions from one extreme to another can keep us unbalanced and in a state of disharmony. That's what we're working with in this exercise.

Visualize the emotions you've identified, and mentally place them at either end of your *tamas–rajas* scales. Notice whether they gather at one or the other end of the scales, and how the weight moves the apparatus up and down as you contemplate one emotion or push away from another. Now draw your attention back from each individual emotion, and experience each one as a part of a larger whole.

Observe your scales and envision that they no longer tip; see them coming into equilibrium. By withdrawing your attachment to the emotions that pull you this way or that, you have found the balance among them. In this place of harmony, you can look at yourself clearly, understand and accept yourself, and move forward in your life. Open your eyes and reflect for a moment on the feelings that came up for you in this exercise.

A Deeper Exploration: Deciding Where to Focus Your Emotional Attention (*Viveka*)

Yoga teaches us how to think clearly. We learn that we are happiest and at our most peaceful when we see things as they are, not as we might want them to be because it serves our own purpose, or because it's convenient. We are also not best served by seeing things the way our inner voices sometime try to convince us we should—with barrages of repetitive judgmental and self-defeating thoughts. Yoga philosophy has a name for this process of looking at yourself clearly, without getting derailed by emotions or shutting down because of them. It is called *viveka*, which can be translated as "true knowledge."[4] When we cultivate *viveka*, we are better able to come away from attachment to emotions by recognizing them for what they are—and what they are not. By developing a discriminating mind, you will understand that your ever-changing emotions are fleeting and that emotional balance lies in your center, where your truth lives.

Sit quietly once more. This time, let a single emotion come into your mind. Notice its tendency to become large, asking for your attention, or perhaps demanding all of it. Without making a judgment about the emotion or trying to "fix" it, see what it would feel like to simply step back from it. Watch it in the same way you might watch a car approaching if you were standing on a sidewalk. You'd first notice the car as a muted noise in the distance. It would become louder as it approached you, and then its sound would fade as it drove away.

How do you imagine you would react to the car? With interest, perhaps, but also with a hint of detachment, knowing that the presence of the car was changing from moment to moment. You'd know the car would come and go, and your mind would use discrimination to recognize that the car wasn't something you needed to get attached to or concerned about. Of course, emotions are much more significant to your mind than a car, yet the image is apt for our practice. When you practice yoga and pay attention to thoughts and emotions—showing interest, but also a hint of detachment—you start to recognize emotions for what they are, fleeting and ever-changing. They are in your mind, but they do not define you. With your yoga practice as a tool and support, you can come into balance amid the constant movement and turmoil of your emotional life. Open your eyes and get ready for your balancing yoga practice.

THREE QUESTIONS TO PREPARE YOU FOR PRACTICE

Before you begin your physical practice, take a moment to reflect on these three questions. Do not judge or overanalyze your responses—merely notice them now, and then return to them after your practice to note any changes you may experience.

1. Visualize your current mood as a set of scales, and imagine that you are holding a stack of weighted discs. How many would you place on the *rajas* and *tamas* sides of the scales? Is one side weighed down by too many discs?
2. Notice your physical posture right now. What, if any, areas of imbalance do you notice?
3. What is one area of your life you feel you manage in a balanced way?

I chose the poses in this practice to help you develop both physical and mental balance. By grounding yourself into the earth, you will bring the far reaches of your body into balance. And by grounding your mind confidently into your body, you will bring your thoughts and emotions closer to your core self, where they can exist in harmony with each other. As you connect all the parts of yourself at this center—the place we first connected to back in Chapter 5—you will find a sense of integration, a unity that becomes a stabilizing, balancing foundation for your life.

YOGA PRACTICE FOR BALANCE

1. Cross-Legged Seated Pose with Ocean Breath

Sit comfortably with your legs crossed on the floor or on a folded blanket, or sit in a chair if you like. Your spine should be long and tall and your chest broad and open. Bring your hands into Prayer Position. For your balancing practice, consider that by bringing your hands to your heart center, you are creating an intention to bring all the parts of yourself into balance. Focusing on your intention during your practice can help to bring you into what the *Yoga Sutras of Patañjali* calls "the state in which activity and silence are equally balanced in the mind."[5] Release your hands and rest them on your thighs in the Gesture of Consciousness.

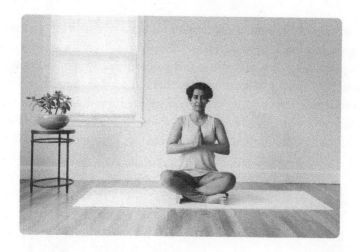

To get ready for a balancing Ocean Breath practice, first notice the length of your breaths in and out. If you are feeling anxious, you may find each breath shallow, you may feel as if you can't get enough air, or you may notice that your inhalations are long but your exhalations are short. If you feel depressed, you may notice an inability to breathe deeply. Observe your breath without judgment, remembering that whatever emotion lies behind your breath is fleeting and impermanent.

Inhale deeply, pause, gently contract your throat muscles, and create an Ocean Breath exhale to begin your practice. Keep your throat muscles contracted and create an Ocean Breath inhale as well. Continue to practice full Ocean Breath, guiding your inhales and exhales into balance. If your inhales are strong and your exhales are weak, focus your attention on your exhales to lengthen them, slowly but surely. Conversely, if your exhales are stronger than your inhales, bring air slowly into your body, from the base of your spine into your abdomen and then into your chest, creating a long path for your inhales. This may take a few minutes, so patience is truly a virtue right now. You may or may not be able to balance your breath fully today, but perhaps you will notice that your emotions become quieter and your mind feels more harmonious, thanks to your efforts to move your breath in a more balanced direction.

2. Boat Pose

Approach this pose by honoring any limitations in your lower back. In the first step, check in with your back to make sure it is comfortable; proceed into the second step only if it is. However you practice, this pose will enhance balance and stability through your hips, uplift and space in your chest, and inner strength in your core.

Sit on your mat with your legs bent and your feet on the floor. Hold the backs of your thighs and lean slightly back until your feet lift up from the floor. Notice whether your back rounds or your chest hollows out. Play with the position of your

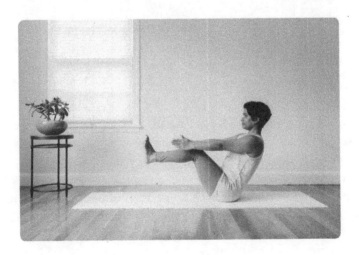

hips until you feel that they are stable and evenly grounded on the floor, enabling you to elongate your torso and broaden your chest. If your back is comfortable, stretch your arms straight forward, with your palms facing each other. Remain in this position for ten to twenty seconds, finding—and rediscovering, if you feel unstable—your physical balance. In moments when you are balanced, observe a quality of quiet clarity in your thoughts.

3. Balancing Sun Salutation

The focus in this Sun Salutation practice is to bring balance into your breath and movements. Start in Mountain Pose with your eyes lowered or closed. Mountain Pose has another name, which is worth considering in this context. In Sanskrit, this name is *samasthiti*, which comes from the root words *sama*, meaning "same," "equal," or "upright," and *sthiti*, meaning "to establish" or "to stand."[6] In this Sun Salutation, set your intention to bring equal effort not only into Mountain Pose, but into every pose. In other words, see if you can move through this flow in a place of physical and mental balance. In each movement, feel your feet equally grounded. Balance the lengths of your breaths and the intensity of your movements, so you can feel a sense of integration as you move through the flow. Practice two rounds of Sun Salutation, and when you are finished, remain in Mountain Pose for an extra few breaths, visualizing your body and mind in harmony.

See pages 172–173 for a photographic Sun Salutation refresher.
Mountain Pose
Upward Hand Pose
Standing Forward Bend Pose
Standing Forward Bend Pose—Head Up
Standing Forward Bend Pose
Downward Facing Dog Pose
High Plank Pose
Four Limb Staff Pose
Cobra Pose or Upward Facing Dog Pose
Downward Facing Dog Pose
Standing Forward Bend Pose
Standing Forward Bend Pose—Head Up

Standing Forward Bend Pose
Upward Hand Pose
Mountain Pose

4. Triangle Pose and Half-Moon Pose

A yoga sequence to help you create balance wouldn't be complete without a balancing standing pose. Half-Moon Pose is a beautiful expression of balance in your physical body and the expansive, uplifting opening of your heart that comes with it. You'll begin by first coming into Triangle Pose, which will give you both the stability and openness to move into Half-Moon Pose.

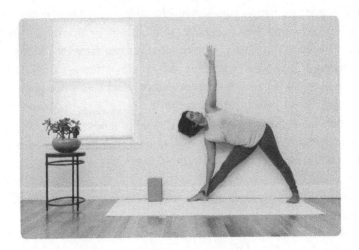

Stand with your feet about four feet apart on your mat, with your back facing a wall and your feet six inches away from the wall. Place a block next to the little toe of your right foot. Turn your left foot slightly inward, and turn your right leg completely out, so your foot is parallel to the wall. Your right knee should be in line with your right ankle. Lift your arms to shoulder height. Hold this position for one deep inhalation, opening your chest completely as you reach your arms apart from each other. Exhaling, bend from your right hip and reach to the right, continuing to stretch your arms straight out. Bring your right hand down onto your lower leg. If you feel comfortable with more stretch, place your hand on your block or on the floor. Reach your left arm upward. Stay in this position, called Triangle Pose, for two breaths, feeling your feet balanced on the earth and experiencing an even stretch through your legs and trunk. Extend from your right hand up through your arms and chest, all the way to your left hand, and feel your heart open and spreading.

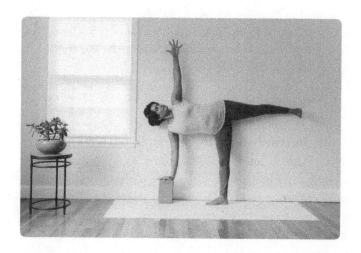

Bend your right knee and take a small step with your left foot toward your right foot, placing your right hand on your block. Lunge forward over your right foot and walk your block forward with your hand. Your right hand should be directly under your right shoulder. Move forward until your left foot lifts off the floor and your left leg swings upward, like the gentle curve of the moon. The first few times you practice this pose, you may like to lean into the wall for support. Once your balance improves, you'll be able to keep your body a few inches away from the wall—knowing it is there for you if you need it. You'll experience the confidence and inner strength that comes from working on physical balance.

Be sure to keep your right foot fully grounded so your right leg remains strong and stable, lifting up toward your hips. Reach your left leg and the crown of your head away from each other, finding a harmonious and balanced feeling of space throughout your body as your left arm extends toward the sky, opening and broadening your heart.

Pause for a moment and consider the qualities of a half-moon. At this time in its monthly cycle, half of the moon is illuminated by the sun, and the other half is in shadow. Although you see only the half that is illuminated, you know that the other half still exists. As the moon and earth rotate, the moon comes into fullness and becomes bright and completely lit. Yoga practice creates a similar synergy in your body as all parts of yourself become illuminated in their own time, so you can see and understand yourself with clarity and harmony.

When you are ready to come out of Half-Moon Pose, bend your right knee, reach your left leg to the left, and place your left foot on the floor. Place your right hand on your right shin and slowly straighten your right leg, coming back into Tri-angle Pose for a moment. Then lift your trunk and arms and turn your feet so they are parallel. Repeat Triangle Pose and Half-Moon Pose on your left side.

5. Restorative Bridge Pose II (with a Block)

Lie on your mat with a block within reach. With your knees bent and your feet firmly planted into the earth, lift your hips and place your block under them. Place the block at the lowest height for a very gentle stretch; turn it to the medium height for a more active stretch; use it at its highest height for even more intensity. Take a moment to check that your lower back is comfortable; adjust the block height so

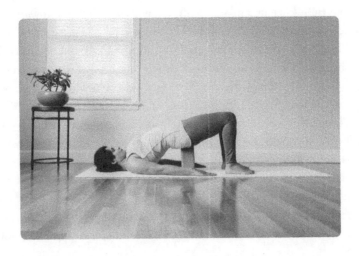

you can remain in the pose for three to five minutes without pain. You should feel balance in several parts of your body: your feet balanced on the floor, your hips balanced on the block, and your shoulders evenly grounded into the earth. Take a moment to feel yourself in this state and notice the quality of your thoughts. Perhaps they become quiet and more balanced as well.

Focus on your diaphragm and chest, experiencing them as lifted and open. Patricia Walden, the Iyengar yoga teacher and mentor to the yoga instructors in our studies, connects an open chest with the ability to see yourself as you truly are, clearly and free from self-judgment. As she puts it, this sort of openness "changes how you perceive the world and how the world perceives you."[7] With your discriminating mind (*viveka*, which we discussed earlier in this chapter), you can feel free to notice the quality of emotions that rise up in Restorative Bridge Pose II. Acknowledge them for what they are—fleeting, changing emotions that do not define you. Stay focused on your true, abiding self, dwelling within your open heart center.

With your chin in a slightly tucked position in this pose, feel the soft vibration of your breath and imagine it massaging your throat. When depression is dominant, feel the vibration of breath reawaken the life-supporting energy in your heart. When you are anxious and your mind is racing, let the vibration be a lullaby that soothes and calms your emotions.

To come out, firm your legs and hips and gently lift your hips off the block. Slowly release your spine onto the earth.

6. Reclining Twist Pose

Lying on your mat, draw your knees into your chest and hug them for a moment. Extend your arms at shoulder height, and as you exhale, allow your knees to fall to your right. You can rest your knees on the floor or support them on a block. Linger in this soft, soothing stretch for a few breaths, turning your trunk and head to the left as you feel your lower back releasing into the stretch. Notice the length and softness through your abdomen and chest. Imagine yourself releasing unhelpful emotions and creating more space in your heart for productive and positive energy. As you do, you may notice your thoughts becoming clearer and more discerning. Inhale as you bring your legs back to center, and repeat the pose on the opposite side. When you are finished, roll to one side and come to a seated position. Take a

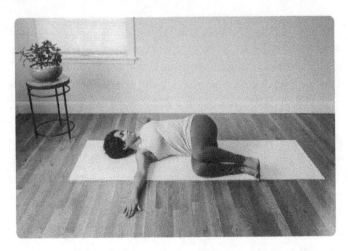

moment to feel the way practicing this pose on one side of your body and then the other brings a sense of balance to your body and mind.

7. Seated Wide-Angle Pose

Sit upright and take your legs wide apart from each other. If this is uncomfortable for you, sit on a folded blanket and bend your knees slightly. Raise your arms and

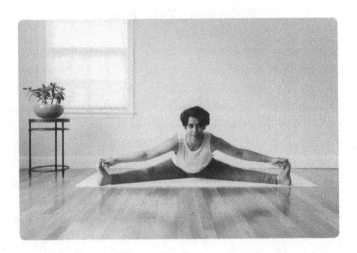

lengthen your trunk upward. As you exhale, fold forward from your hips and hold your feet, or hold each foot with a belt. Keep your neck long and gaze softly forward or downward. Notice the sensations in your legs and back. You should feel a comfortable and sustainable stretch, but if you feel strain, bend your knees until your body is happy.

Stay in the pose for a few breaths. Let your mind draw inward and notice that as the sensations in your body change, your thoughts change as well. Moment to moment, watch your thoughts coming away from the poles of depression and anxiety, into a place of inner balance, as you remain grounded between your equally stretching legs.

8. Balancing Inverted Pose

Set yourself up in Inverted Pose by sitting with your side against a wall, lying down, and swinging your legs up the wall. Slide a bolster under your hips to come into the pose. Add a blanket if you enjoy more height. Notice that your trunk, neck, and head are in a position similar to how they were in Restorative Bridge Pose II—your trunk is long, and your diaphragm and chest are broad and open. As you practice this pose,

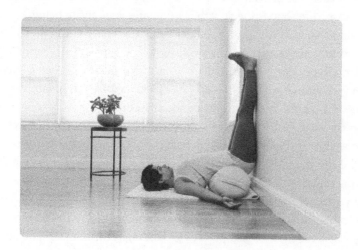

visualize your heart center—*Anahata chakra*, your seat of emotions. Recall that the heart center is literally at the center of your *chakras*; there are three below it and three above it. In your body—in your life—your heart center is the ever-steady still point. It is the place of fortitude and equanimity that helps you create and sustain your balance.

9. Plow Pose and Shoulder Stand

After you have practiced Inverted Pose for some time and your body is very comfortable in an inverted position, you can practice Shoulder Stand—sometimes called Shoulder Balance Pose—for a deeper inversion experience. Shoulder Stand is more rigorous than Inverted Pose and asks more of your physical body in terms of supporting its own weight. Thus, it is contraindicated for many shoulder, back, and neck issues, eye and ear conditions, and brain injuries. We advised you to consult your medical doctor before beginning any yoga practice; please specifically consult your provider before you practice this pose.

Shoulder Stand is a pose that can "turn your world upside down" in very positive ways. Many students find that as they practice it, they gain new insights and perspectives that greatly help with challenging emotions and everyday life situations. In this upside-down balance pose, your arms and shoulders become your solid ground, while the rest of your body becomes light and lifts upward. Your breath becomes a strong life-supporting flow that stimulates your entire being.

You'll start your journey into Shoulder Stand by first coming into Plow Pose. Because your feet are resting on the wall, Plow Pose gives you a more supported upside-down experience than Shoulder Stand. Stack three folded blankets and place them on your mat with the folded edges facing a wall—start with the blankets about two feet from the wall, or a little more if your legs are very long. Sit facing the wall on the edge of the blankets. Adjust the placement of the blankets so your feet are flat against the wall when you stretch out your legs straight. Turn your body around 180 degrees, and lie down with your arms and shoulders on the blankets and your head on your mat. The crown of your head will be facing the wall. As you exhale, bend your knees, swing your legs up over your head, and take your feet to the wall. Place your hands on your back and straighten your legs. You are now in Plow Pose. Linger here for a few breaths, evenly grounding your shoulders and upper arms into your supports as you lift up through your trunk.

When you are ready, take one leg away from the wall and stretch it straight up toward the ceiling. If that feels comfortable, follow it with the other leg. With both

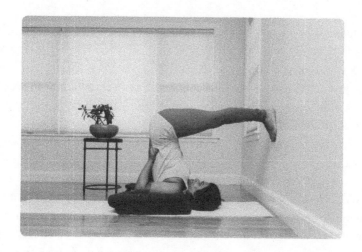

legs lifting toward the sky, you are now in Shoulder Stand. Your breath should be smooth and even, and your eyes should be soft. If you feel discomfort in your neck, come out of Shoulder Stand and practice Inverted Pose instead.

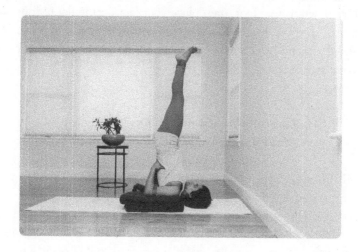

For extra support in Plow Pose and Shoulder Stand, you can use a belt to stabilize your arms (pictured above). Make a belt into a loop about the same width as your shoulders. When you lie down on your blankets, place the belt around one of your arms, just above your elbow, keeping the belt close to your body. Once you lift your legs and bring your feet to the wall in Plow Pose, slip the belt onto your other arm, just above the elbow. Take your hands onto your back then proceed into Shoulder Stand. You should feel well-grounded through your upper arms and feel a nice sense of lift through your trunk.

Stay in Shoulder Stand for about twenty seconds in the beginning, and gradually increase the time as you continue to practice the pose. As you explore yourself in this upside-down, balanced position, use your discriminating mind to notice all that is happening inside, especially your ever-changing thoughts and emotions. Be interested in the emotions that come up, yet notice the sense of equanimity that also arises, so you can be present to your emotions without feeling overwhelmed by or overly attached to them. Notice that your thoughts and feelings come and go, yet you can remain balanced, both physically and mentally. Perhaps you will discover a new approach to a vexing everyday issue, or perhaps you will realize the power that lies within you, the life-supporting energy that can create and maintain emotional harmony.

When you are ready to come down, bring your feet back to the wall in Plow Pose. If you are using a belt around your arms, slip it off. Bend your knees and gently roll your hips down to the floor, then place your feet on the floor. Shift your body toward the wall so you can rest for a few moments with your hips on the blankets, and your shoulders and head on the floor. Then roll over onto your side and come up into a comfortable seated position.

10. Deep Relaxation with Ocean Breath— Your Harmonious, Balanced Mind

Place a folded blanket near the top of your mat. Sit on your mat with your knees bent, feet resting on the floor. Place a bolster under your knees. Place your hands behind you on the floor. Press your hands down and lift your chest, then slowly lie down, feeling your hips, back, and shoulders balanced on and supported by the ground. Support your head on the folded blanket. Feel your knees balanced on your bolster, and the weight of your heels equally resting on your mat.

Visualize yourself standing at the edge of a beautiful ocean, watching the waves. Notice how each wave flows up along the shore, seems to pause in a peaceful

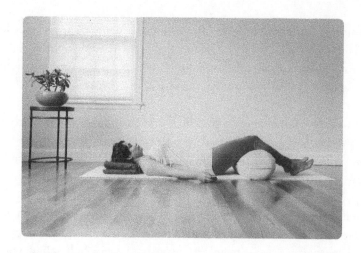

moment of stillness, and then gently retreats as it flows back into the sea. Observe the waves with interest, yet with the understanding that nature can find its balance on its own—you don't need to do anything except be present to each wave, to each moment, as you honor nature's cycles of balance.

Inhale normally, gently contract your throat muscles, and begin Ocean Breath on your exhalation. If you are comfortable doing so, practice full Ocean Breaths, creating the sound of an inner sigh both when you inhale and when you exhale. Imagine your breathing follows the rhythm of the ocean's waves. Just as a wave starts at a distance from the shore, feel your inhalation gently rising from the base of your spine. As the wave crests and flows onto the shore, let your breath rise into your diaphragm and pool around your heart. Notice a moment of silence at the top of the wave, your heart filled with nature's healing, balancing energy and your mind soothed. As the wave quietly recedes into the ocean, feel your exhale quietly releasing outward into the earth. Breath by breath, notice how your breathing comes into balance, your thoughts moving away from the emotional fluctuations of depression and anxiety into a place of clarity, harmony, and balance. After five or six rounds, release your Ocean Breath and take a couple of normal breaths in and out.

You are now ready to move into your twenty-minute Coherent Breathing practice. Aim for a six-second inhale and a six-second exhale. Just let your breath flow in an even, balanced way. Even though you're no longer contracting your throat muscles, continue to visualize your inhales like the ocean waves gently flowing along the shore of your body, bringing in fresh, life-sustaining energy. See your exhales softly ebbing and receding back into space, taking along unneeded thoughts and emotions.

After your Coherent Breathing practice, reflect for a moment on the three questions you carried with you into your practice.

1. Are you more aware of what your body and mind need to come into balance?
2. Briefly scan your body. Where do you feel a sense of balance?
3. Can you imagine how your practice can help you be more balanced in your approach to one particular area of your life?

As you finish this last of our five practice chapters, feel how far you have come on your journey. Perhaps you can find that along with balance, calm, energy, empowerment, and centeredness, you are able to understand your whole self in a new way.

LOOKING AHEAD WITH HOPE AND CONFIDENCE

We began our journey together with a reflection on the courage required to take even the smallest step toward emotional health. I'd like to come back to that idea now as we look back on the road we've traveled so far—and as we look ahead to your whole future.

"Courage is a heart word," says the writer and researcher Brené Brown. "The root of the word courage is *cor*—the Latin word for heart. In one of its earliest forms, the word courage meant 'To speak one's mind by telling all one's heart.'"[1]

Throughout this book, I've talked about the yogic philosophy that encourages (emphasis on *courage*) you to connect with your heart, and all that lies within it.

What does courage mean? In our everyday context, it often means willingness to face something frightening or difficult, from a soldier being called to war to a pregnant woman anticipating labor and delivery. But to me, emotional courage lies within yourself, rather than being a place or a situation that calls for your attention.

Making lasting changes to your emotions asks that you look inward and find the courage to closely examine what you see. It requires the tenacity to stay present to whatever you find there, as uncomfortable and painful as your emotions may feel, and to hold them and care for them with love and compassion. Self-acceptance is at the core of self-understanding—and that in turn leads to self-transformation.

Undertaking this journey toward wellness, toward wholeness, requires profound bravery. The stakes are high. But the rewards are great. As you continue the healing work we have begun together, you are more likely to feel those benefits in your daily life.

FOUR WAYS TO SUPPORT YOUR ONGOING EMOTIONAL GROWTH

In this book, you have explored different ways yoga can deepen how you discover yourself, connect with yourself, and care for yourself in times of depression or anxiety. You've undertaken this work with the courage you needed to summon, the courage to face yourself exactly as you are, the courage to ask yourself to take one step at a time toward wellness and wholeness.

Now that you know you have this deep inner reserve of courage and wisdom, and now that you know how yoga can serve your life, you might find yourself wondering how you can continue to support your emotional growth when you are not "on the mat."

In other words, how can you integrate yoga into the larger picture of your journey toward wellness? Fostering emotional health is a lifelong endeavor that each of us undertakes in our own way. I like to think that these four ideas connect with a yogic outlook, a view of both your inner life and the world around you that is rooted in the idea that everything is connected and has the potential to propel us toward balance, alignment, and wholeness.

Spend Time in Nature

The emotional impact of being outdoors or connected to nature is of such interest to scientists that it has emerged as its own field of research called ecopsychology.[2]

Studies have shown that taking a walk in an urban park can improve your mood more than taking the same type of walk in a built-up city setting.[3] Other research has shown that simply listening to the sounds of nature, through an app or even using a white noise machine, can promote measurable relaxation and well-being.[4]

How does this connect with your yoga practice? We've discussed throughout this book the yogic idea that everything in the universe displays some combination of inertia, activity, and harmony (*tamas*, *rajas*, and *sattva*, if you need a refresher). Taking this idea out into the natural world can enrich your sense of connection to rocks, trees, flowers, clouds, rivers, insects, animals—everything you notice in any outdoor space.

Some people enjoy practicing yoga outdoors, but you don't need to be doing poses to have a yogic experience of nature. The next time you are in a natural space, whether in your backyard or a neighborhood park, on a beach or a hiking trail, be mindful of the energy that's all around you—and look for ways you can take in whatever you need to improve your mood in that moment. If you're feeling ungrounded, sitting beneath a tree may help you find your roots. When you feel tight and stuck from depression, take a walk where you can see the horizon, whether it's at the ocean, in an open field, or on a hilltop. Let yourself expand into the spaciousness around you. When you feel overwhelmed by your overactive mind, follow Eckhart Tolle's advice to "Look at a tree, a flower, a plant. Let your awareness rest upon it. How still they are, how deeply rooted in Being. Allow nature to teach you stillness."[5]

Use Ocean Breath and Coherent Breathing Throughout Your Day

In each yoga practice in this book, you spent time practicing Ocean Breath and Coherent Breathing, the slow intentional breaths that signal your brain to come into restful balance. Breath practices are perhaps the most "portable" of all the practices we've done together—you can use them at almost any time, in any physical or emotional place you may find yourself, to effectively reset your state of mind. Some best times to practice yogic breathing may be during downtimes in your day, such as commuting to work or school on public transportation, between daily tasks, or during a lunch break. And they are especially helpful when you're preparing to take a catnap during the day or going to sleep at night.

It's important to spend dedicated time practicing Ocean Breath or Coherent Breathing; twenty-minute sessions are ideal for the latter. But once you have learned the technique, very short sessions can also have a positive impact on your mood, if for no other reason than serving as a reminder that you have a deep well of strength to draw on as you navigate your day. Richard Brown and Patricia Gerbarg, in *The Healing Power of the Breath*, say the more you practice Coherent Breathing, "the better you will feel." They add, "Do as much as you like to prevent a buildup of stress and to relieve anxiety."[6]

So if you are standing at the bus stop or sitting in a waiting room at the doctor's office and feel your anxiety level rising, even ten rounds of Ocean Breath or Coherent Breathing can help quiet your racing mind. If you are at a dinner party and find yourself ruminating on your personal relationships or lacking the energy to engage in conversation, those same ten breaths can shore up your reserves, helping you come back to yourself and remember all that you have to contribute.

Breath practices aren't appropriate at all times of the day, though. When you are engaged in an activity that requires acute mental attention and quick reflexive actions, such as driving, your mind needs to be focused on the activity, rather than on your breath. But when you are stopped in a traffic jam or at a red light, you can use even a single breath to cue yourself to release tension and calm your nerves.

Remember to Rest

As yoga becomes increasingly popular in the United States, it seems that a new form of yoga practice debuts almost daily. Depending on the source, there are anywhere from eight to fifty major methods of yoga, and that number is likely to continue to climb. As much as different yoga methods vary, something most of them have in common is that practices end with Deep Relaxation, an intentional opportunity for the body and mind to come into a place of profound rest. In a position of total comfort, your body can release tension, and your mind can turn inward. You can honor your body and mind for all the physical and emotional work you have done in your practice—and for the duration of your relaxation, let go of obstacles to your well-being and rest in the calmness of your heart.

It's healthy and important to prioritize rest in your life outside your yoga practice as well. This includes sleep—the Centers for Disease Control and Prevention recommends adults get at least seven hours of sleep per night.[7] For some people, practicing restorative yoga postures, Ocean Breath, or Coherent Breathing right before bed is the recipe for a peaceful night of sleep. The Ocean Breath you first learned in this book, with a normal, long inhale and an Ocean Breath exhale, may be particularly helpful as a sleep aid. You might also want to turn to the calming practice in Chapter 8 and see if it encourages rest for you.

But "rest" does not have to mean "sleep." Just as you do in your yoga practice, look for opportunities to find a quiet moment following any active period in your day. This will help you process any emotions that come up during busy times, and it will create the restorative space you need to transition to the next thing your day may be asking of you.

Reach Out for Support

When you feel frenzied by anxiety or weighed down by depression, one of the most common emotional responses is isolation, a sense that you are struggling alone. Built into yoga philosophy is the idea that though we each work within our own minds and bodies, we are also part of a caring community that can be a source of support in difficult times. "Sometimes, each person's load can only be taken collectively," the Kundalini yoga master Yogi Bhajan said.[8]

Though depression or anxiety might make reaching out for help challenging or even frightening, there are numerous ways to do so. A conversation with your doctor, a therapist, or a counselor can help you connect your emotions to specific conditions that can be treated. Calling or writing to trusted friends or family members can boost your mood and remind you that you are part of a larger community of people who care about you. Even a simple social media post to the effect of "I could use some love today" will likely leave you feeling surrounded by positive energy.

If you decide to expand your practice from your home into a yoga studio, look for a teacher who can help you feel safe and supported in class. I want to offer a special word of encouragement here: it can take some time to find a yoga community that feels like a good fit for you. I suggest you try out a number of local yoga studios and teachers, since each studio and teacher has a particular approach to yoga practice, and many different kinds of classes are offered. Don't give up. One day, a teacher or a particular class will resonate with you, and you will feel supported and welcomed into the group. Keep going back to that teacher or class as often as you can, even when you feel your depression or anxiety flaring or weighing you down.

It can be difficult to ask for help, or even leave your home to go to a class, when you are feeling anxious or depressed. Remember that the gift of yoga practice—the ability to change your emotions and your mind—is not only meant for when you're feeling capable or in a relatively upbeat mood. It is meant to help you lift yourself up in times of deep suffering and need, so that you can feel encouraged and empowered, and fully in relationship with yourself and your life. My hope is that this book might be a lasting way for you to receive this gift, and that you can take what you've learned here into a yoga class that serves your life and bolsters your emotional health.

Counselors, therapists, or therapeutic support groups, whether in person or online, can also be helpful in understanding your emotional challenges in context. Please see the Further Reading and Resources section for tips on how to get started choosing a yoga therapist.

You are not alone—and I mean that literally. Remember that more than one in five American adults experiences a mood disorder at some point in their lives. You have learned a lot about yourself in your work throughout this book. With courage and confidence, you can reach out into the world and expect to find sources of love and support, wherever you are in your journey.

YOUR WHOLE EMOTIONAL LIFE

Wholeness is a theme we've addressed in different ways throughout this book. Yoga philosophy is replete with examples of wholes comprised of various parts—to name only one, the seven *chakras* each hold portions of the totality of energy that dwells within each of us. In science, by contrast, there is no such thing as a "whole" body of research—there are always more questions to ask, more ideas to test, and more to learn.

What about your emotional life? What are the parts of that whole, and what does it mean to live a complete life? I chose the emotional attributes we've explored in this book—centeredness, empowerment, energy, calm, and balance—specifically because I felt they cover the fullness of emotional experiences you may be seeking in your journey through depression or anxiety. Let's briefly review each of these to recall their place in your whole emotional life.

Centeredness

Your center is a safe and grounded place. It is relatively easy to connect the idea of "centering" to your physical body, but with practice it will also become recognizable to you as the source of deep peace and wisdom within yourself. When you access your true center, you meet your authentic self.

Empowerment

Bringing the fullness of your inner strength to a place you can easily access is the feeling of empowerment. Crucial to your ability to manage depression, anxiety, or other life challenges is confidence in your personal power and investment in your ability to face your daily life and navigate everything it asks of you.

Energy

The weight of depression can slow you down, tugging at the motivation you would otherwise summon to embrace each day. Discovering a well of energy within your body, mind, and heart can awaken you to your own potential and remind you of everything you have to contribute to your life.

Calm

Wherever you are in your journey, learning to trust in your ability to become calm and peaceful is a meaningful part of your healing path. In a state of calmness, your mind can slow down enough to become mindfully focused on itself, your emotional state, and what you need to rest and restore your body and mind.

Balance

The point of balance between two opposing forces is a powerful space to inhabit. Whether you're seeking to balance the negative and positive impulses of your natural outlook on the world, or whether you're looking for the balance between activity and rest that is sustainable and healthful for you, balance is a worthy goal.

What came up for you as you reviewed these attributes? You might have felt insecure about how one or more of them still challenge you. You might have noticed progress you've made on others. Or you might also be thinking, "There's so much more to my emotional life than those five qualities." Any of those responses is appropriate and helpful in encouraging you to emerge from this book bolstered by a commitment to integrate yoga into a holistic view of your life and health.

But as you contemplate the role of yoga in your whole emotional life, it's helpful to remember that "wholeness" does not mean "perfection." The "journey toward becoming whole again," which we first discussed in Chapter 1, is not the quest for absolute happiness or constant joy. Instead, it's the mindful orientation of your life toward balance among all the myriad emotions that make your mind the marvelous, complex phenomenon that it is. Remember how yoga philosopher Sally Kempton urges us to pursue "steady effort in the direction you want to go?"[9] Living your whole emotional life means living in honest connection with the obstacles that challenge you, facing your full range of emotions with clear-eyed attention, and bravely putting one foot in front of the other in measured, consistent pursuit of improvement, growth, and progress. You can do this—my years of experience as a yoga teacher combined with my work on Dr. Streeter's studies tells me so.

MEDITATION: YOUR COURAGEOUS HEART

Now let's turn our attention back to your heart, and its brilliant courage. Find a comfortable seat and close your eyes, either completely or halfway. Draw your attention inward toward your heart, so you can be receptive to the messages it needs to tell you.

Visualize your heart center. Recall how in yoga philosophy, an eight-petaled lotus flower sits there, with its bud closed and pointed downward. Through yoga practice, that lotus of the heart comes into bloom.[10] Your ongoing work on and off the mat waters and nourishes your lotus. Your courage empowers it to open at just the right time.

As you breathe normally, visualize the beautiful bud, quietly and patiently abiding its closed position, waiting to be opened as you move into your journey toward healing and self-understanding. Inhale softly and deeply into your heart center, and exhale from your heart center outward through your entire body.

Breath by breath, visualize the bud steadily turning upward and opening into a full, mature bloom, cupping and holding the energy of your heart. Visualize a bright light in the center of the open, luminous lotus flower. See its brave and brilliant light illuminate all that exists within your heart, shedding light on your emotions. Let it brighten how you view yourself and the world around you so you can stay present, even to very strong emotions, and come into self-understanding.

The light of the heart is a constant source of both illumination and courage—to see your emotions, stay with them, and, ultimately, understand and accept them. This light, this courage, is always available to you as a source of support on your healing journey. For the next few moments, just bask in the power of the light of your heart and its ability to help you.

When you are ready to end your meditation, thank your heart for its bravery, its strength, and its tenacity as it continues to be your life-supporting source of courage.

APPENDIX A

Full Practice Sequences

O nce you feel comfortable enough with the five practices that you don't need to refer to the instructions each time, you can step onto your mat and refer to these photographic sequences to cue yourself.

Chapter 5: Center

Your center is a safe and grounded place. It is relatively easy to connect the idea of "centering" to your physical body, but with practice it will also become recognizable to you as the source of deep peace and wisdom within yourself. When you access your true center, you meet your authentic self.

I. Cross-Legged Seated Pose with Ocean Breath >

2. Seated Upward Hand Pose >

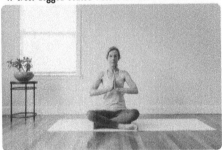 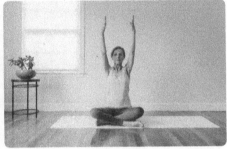

3. Centering Sun Salutation

    Mountain Pose
    Upward Hand Pose
    Standing Forward Bend Pose
    Standing Forward Bend Pose——Head Up
    Standing Forward Bend Pose
    Downward Facing Dog Pose
    High Plank Pose
    Four Limb Staff Pose
    Cobra Pose or Upward Facing Dog Pose
    Downward Facing Dog Pose
    Standing Forward Bend Pose
    Standing Forward Bend Pose——Head Up
    Standing Forward Bend Pose
    Upward Hand Pose
    Mountain Pose

4. Tree Pose >

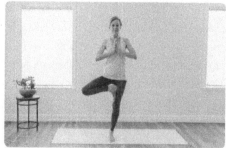

5. Restorative Bridge Pose I (with a Bolster) >

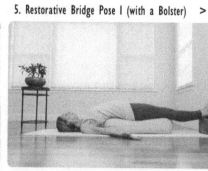

6. Child's Pose—Side Stretch Variation >

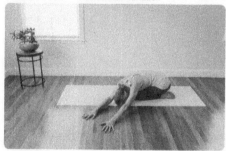

7. Supported Child's Pose Forward Bend >

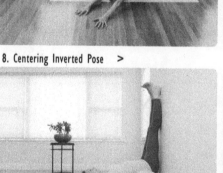

8. Centering Inverted Pose >

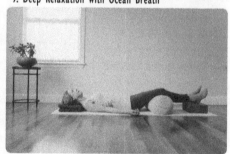

9. Deep Relaxation with Ocean Breath

Chapter 6: Empower

Bringing the fullness of your inner strength to a place you can easily access is the feeling of empowerment. Confidence in your personal power and investment in your ability to face your daily life and navigate everything it asks of you are crucial to your ability to manage depression, anxiety, or other life challenges.

1. Cross-Legged Seated Pose with Ocean Breath **>**

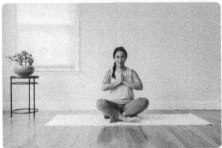

2. Hero's Pose with Upward Bound Knuckle Pose **>**

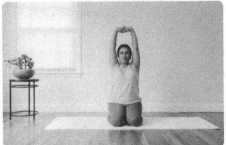

3. Empowering Sun Salutation

Mountain Pose
Upward Hand Pose
Standing Forward Bend Pose
Standing Forward Bend Pose—Head Up
Standing Forward Bend Pose
Downward Facing Dog Pose
High Plank Pose
Four Limb Staff Pose
Cobra Pose or Upward Facing Dog Pose
Downward Facing Dog Pose
Standing Forward Bend Pose
Standing Forward Bend Pose—Head Up
Standing Forward Bend Pose
Upward Hand Pose
Mountain Pose

4. Warrior I >

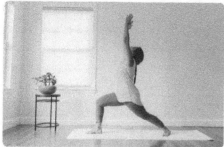

5. Supported Reclining Backbend Pose >

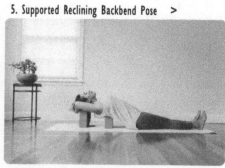

6. Reclining Bent Knee Twist >

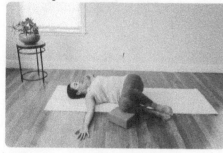

7. Head-to-Knee Pose >

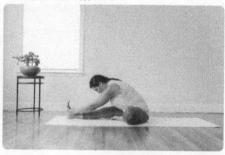

8. Empowering Inverted Pose >

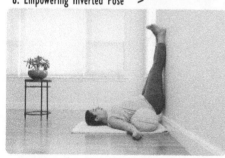

9. Deep Relaxation with Ocean Breath

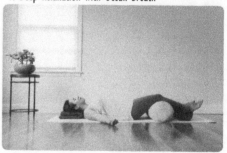

Chapter 7: Energize

The weight of depression can slow you down, tugging at the motivation you would otherwise summon to embrace each day. Discovering a well of energy within your body, mind, and heart can awaken you to your own potential and remind you of everything you have to contribute to your life.

I. Cross-Legged Seated Pose with Ocean Breath   >

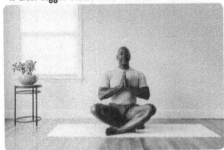

2. Hero's Pose with Cow-Face Arms   >

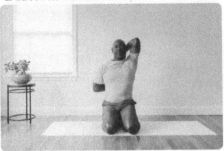

3. Energizing Sun Salutation

    Mountain Pose
    Upward Hand Pose
    Standing Forward Bend Pose
    Standing Forward Bend Pose—Head Up
    Standing Forward Bend Pose
    Downward Facing Dog Pose
    High Plank Pose
    Four Limb Staff Pose
    Cobra Pose or Upward Facing Dog Pose
    Downward Facing Dog Pose
    Standing Forward Bend Pose
    Standing Forward Bend Pose—Head Up
    Standing Forward Bend Pose
    Upward Hand Pose
    Mountain Pose

4. Warrior II >

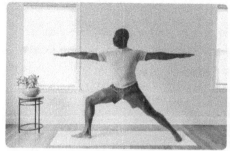

5. Bridge Pose >

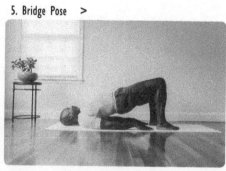

6. Marichi's Twist I >

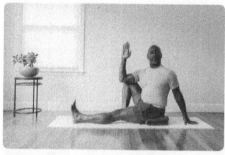

7. Seated Forward Bend Pose >

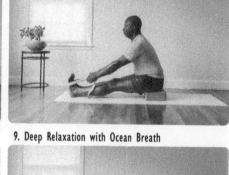

8. Energizing Inverted Pose >

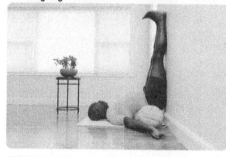

9. Deep Relaxation with Ocean Breath

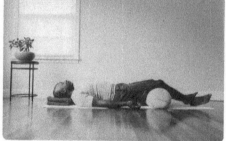

Chapter 8: Calm

Wherever you are in your journey, learning to trust in your ability to become calm and peaceful is a meaningful part of your healing path. In a state of calmness, your mind can slow down enough to become mindfully focused on yourself, your emotional state, and what you need to rest and restore your body and mind.

I. Cross-Legged Seated Pose with Ocean Breath   >

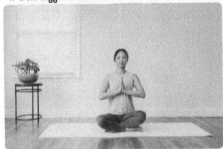

2. Reclining Hand-to-Big-Toe Poses I and II   >

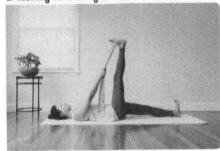 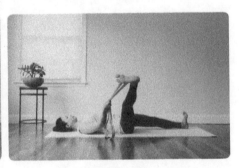

3. Calming Sun Salutation

Mountain Pose
Upward Hand Pose
Standing Forward Bend Pose
Standing Forward Bend Pose—
   Head Up
Standing Forward Bend Pose
Downward Facing Dog Pose
High Plank Pose
Four Limb Staff Pose

Cobra Pose or Upward
   Facing Dog Pose
Downward Facing Dog Pose
Standing Forward Bend Pose
Standing Forward Bend Pose—
   Head Up
Standing Forward Bend Pose
Upward Hand Pose
Mountain Pose

4. Wide-Legged Standing Forward Bend Pose   >

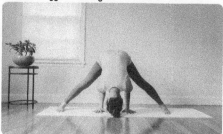

5. Standing Backbend Pose   >

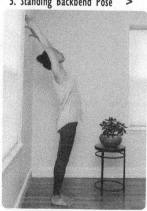

6. Reclining Bound Angle Pose   >

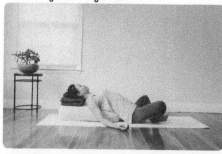

7. Child's Pose   >

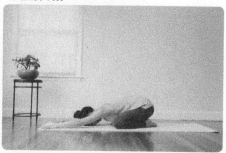

8. Seated Forward Bend Pose with Head Supported   >

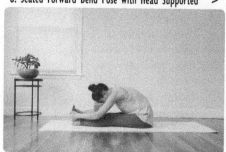

9. Calming Inverted Pose   >

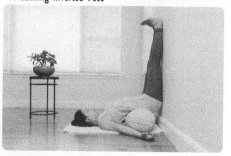

10. Deep Relaxation with Ocean Breath

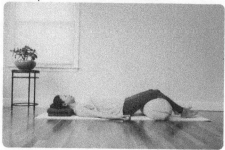

Chapter 9: Balance

The point of balance between two opposing forces is a powerful space to inhabit. Whether you're seeking to balance the negative and positive impulses of your natural outlook on the world, or whether you're looking for the balance between activity and rest that is sustainable and healthful for you, balance is a worthy goal.

---

1. Cross-Legged Seated Pose with Ocean Breath   >

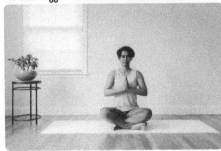

2. Boat Pose   >

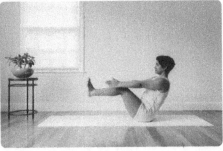

3. Balancing Sun Salutation

Mountain Pose
Upward Hand Pose
Standing Forward Bend Pose
Standing Forward Bend Pose—
  Head Up
Standing Forward Bend Pose
Downward Facing Dog Pose
High Plank Pose
Four Limb Staff Pose

Cobra Pose or Upward
  Facing Dog Pose
Downward Facing Dog Pose
Standing Forward Bend Pose
Standing Forward Bend Pose—
  Head Up
Standing Forward Bend Pose
Upward Hand Pose
Mountain Pose

4. Triangle Pose and Half-Moon Pose   >

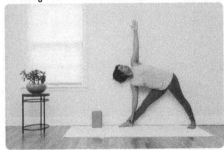

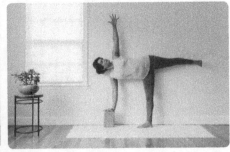

5. Restorative Bridge Pose II (with a Block) >

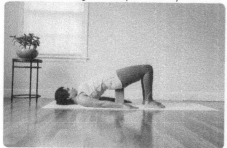

6. Reclining Twist Pose >

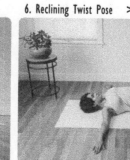

7. Seated Wide-Angle Pose >

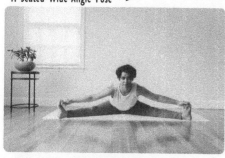

8. Balancing Inverted Pose >

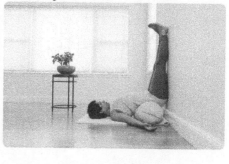

9. Plow Pose and Shoulder Stand >

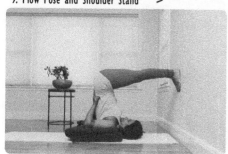

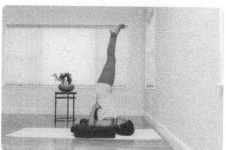

10. Deep Relaxation with Ocean Breath

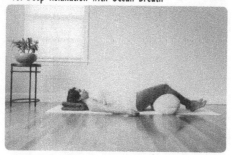

APPENDIX B

Sun Salutation Sequence

S un Salutation is included in each of the five practices in this book. You can refer to page 42 for detailed instructions on how to practice this flow. Once you're familiar with it, you can refer to these photos as a quick guide.

Mountain Pose >

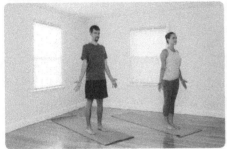

Upward Hand Pose >

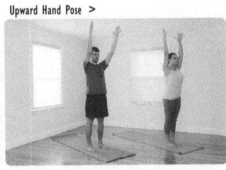

Standing Forward Bend Pose >

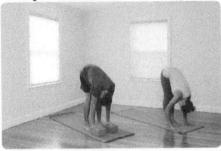

Standing Forward Bend Pose—Head Up >

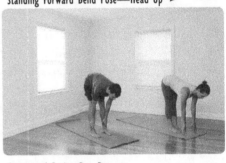

Standing Forward Bend Pose >

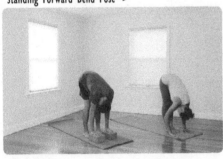

Downward Facing Dog Pose >

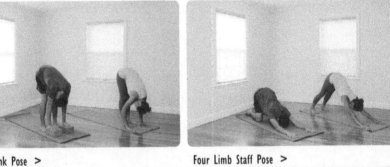

High Plank Pose >

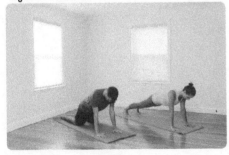

Four Limb Staff Pose >

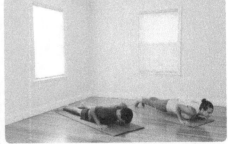

Cobra Pose or Upward Facing Dog Pose >

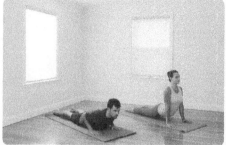

Downward Facing Dog Pose >

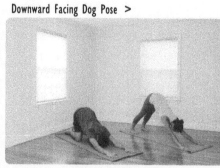

Standing Forward Bend Pose >

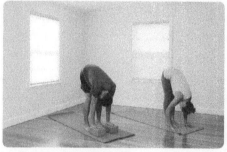

Standing Forward Bend Pose—Head Up >

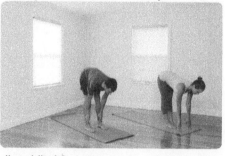

Standing Forward Bend Pose >

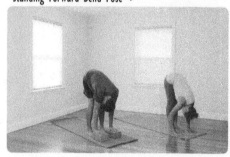

Upward Hand Pose >

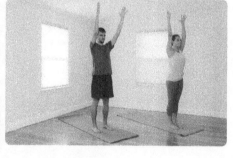

Mountain Pose

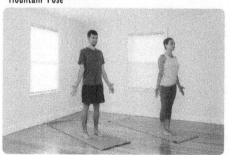

ACKNOWLEDGMENTS

Creating a book is as daunting a process as it is an exciting one. Many people supported this book from its infancy, and now, as it passes from our hands into yours, we are overflowing with gratitude and appreciation for each person who helped it reach you.

First, we'd like to thank those who helped us create the part of the book that you read. Our agent, Ryan Harbage, believed in us and in our idea, and his guidance helped us navigate the publishing world with confidence and enthusiasm. Our team at Lifelong Books has served as just that—a team that's been here to support and encourage us at every stage of the process. Renée Sedliar, our astounding editor, made the manuscript sharper and smarter—and her positivism kept us inspired and excited throughout the writing period. The editorial group at Lifelong, including assistant editor Miriam Riad, project editor Michael Clark, copyeditor Beth Partin, and everyone else at Hachette Books/Lifelong, was supportive, responsive, and just plain kind. Mareshia Donald, PhD, generously read an early draft of the manuscript, and her comments helped us meet readers where they are while respecting the rigor expected by the scientific community. The contributions of Chris C. Streeter, MD, to this work can't be overstated. She was a careful and thoughtful reader of multiple drafts, and her patient explanations of complex scientific concepts enriched both our understanding and our writing. We also must seize the opportunity to thank her for her groundbreaking research and curious mind, without which this book would simply not exist.

Reflecting on the research, we acknowledge the many dedicated Iyengar yoga teachers whose time and contributions strengthened our studies at Boston University School of Medicine (BUSM). Thank you to Carol Faulkner, Marysia Gensler,

Mary Wixted, Cathy Mann, Jean Stawarz, Annie Hoffman, Nancy Turnquist, and Lynnae LeBlanc.

Many thanks are also due to the research staff at the Boston Yoga Research Center at BUSM—Anne Marie Hernon, Greylin Nielsen, Maren Nyer, PhD, Jennifer Johnston, PhD, and Tammy Scott, PhD—for their tireless work over long hours to ensure that all the technical and scientific requirements of the studies run smoothly and correctly. They create such a welcoming, supportive environment for those with depression and anxiety.

We must also note with gratitude that the funding for Dr. Streeter's studies was provided by R21AT004014 and R01AT007483 (CCS), M01RR00533 (Boston University Clinical and Translational Science Institute), and U11RR025771 (General Clinical Research Unit at Boston University Medical Center).

Now, on to thanks to those who created the part of the book you see. Alex Camlin and Amy Quinn designed a gorgeous cover and book layout. Tracy Rodriguez's clear, creative photographic eye inspired us at every turn, and we are so proud to have her images grace these pages. Our yoga models were so generous with both their time and their skills—Janet DeVasher (Center), Eleonora Cordovani (Empower), Jeffrey Thomas (Energize), Aya Mishina (Calm), and Sunetra Banerjee (Balance) truly embodied the emotional attributes featured in their respective chapters. The wonderful brother-and-sister team of Maggie and Cole Chadwick brought cheerful and playful energy to their Sun Salutation sequences. Maura Conron created the elegant illustration of the *chakras* and *nadis*. Thanks are also due to Addie Dublin for sharing her extraordinary potted plant collection with us, bringing even more life into our photos. We are also grateful to Mira Whiting for coaxing out our inner warmth on a chilly day for our author photos.

Finally, a word of acknowledgment from each of us individually.

From Liz:

I begin by thanking Holly Lebowitz Rossi for our extraordinary relationship in yoga and writing. Holly, your quick, inquisitive, and thoughtful intellect lifts me up to places I never expect to reach. Your light guides the way through each writing journey. Your fortitude and conviction remained through all that came our way . . . and it wasn't always an easy journey. I offer one thousand and eight *pranams* to you. I also thank each and every yoga practitioner whom I have had the honor of teaching; you are the real teachers. To Patricia Walden, I thank you for your ever-present light, your depth, and your astute guidance for our team of yoga teachers throughout the studies. To my husband and daughter, Peter and Ryah Belford, thank you for your abiding presence in my life.

From Holly:

I am lucky enough to be entering my second decade of connection with the incomparable Liz Owen. Liz, I've learned from you that there is strength and flexibility within me, that I do not have to abide discomfort, and that there is almost always an adjustment I can make that will help me take one more step in the direction of alignment, growth, and confidence. Those lessons have reverberated through my life, as they live in this book. Thank you for being my teacher, friend, and role model. I would also like to thank the community of friends, neighbors, family members, and others who have helped me care for my own emotional health. Your love and support surrounded me as I worked on this book—and far beyond. Finally, my husband, Rob, and son, Ben, moved mountains (and furniture, and schedules, and mealtimes) to allow me the space to complete this project. I love you both so very much.

FURTHER READING AND RESOURCES

B elow is a selection of books and other resources that may be helpful in expanding your connection to yoga for depression and anxiety, exploring related practices to bring your moods into balance, and deepening your knowledge of general yoga practice and philosophy.

Yoga and Mental Health—Depression, Anxiety, and PTSD

Emerson, David. *Trauma-Sensitive Yoga in Therapy: Bringing the Body into Treatment*. New York: W. W. Norton, 2015.

Emerson, David, and Elizabeth Hopper, PhD. *Overcoming Trauma Through Yoga: Reclaiming Your Body*. Berkeley, CA: North Atlantic Books, 2011.

Forbes, Bo. *Yoga for Emotional Balance: Simple Practices to Help Relieve Anxiety and Depression*. Boston: Shambhala, 2011.

Helbert, Karla. *Yoga for Grief and Loss: Poses, Meditation, Devotion, Self-Reflection, Selfless Acts, Ritual*. London: Singing Dragon, 2016.

Mason, Heather, and Kelly Birch. *Yoga for Mental Health*. Edinburgh: Handspring Publishing, 2018.

Miller, Richard C., PhD. *The iRest Program for Healing PTSD: A Proven-Effective Approach to Using Yoga Nidra Meditation and Deep Relaxation Techniques to Overcome Trauma*. Oakland, CA: New Harbinger Publications, Inc., 2015.

Sausys, Antonio. *Yoga for Grief Relief: Simple Practices for Transforming Your Grieving Mind and Body*. Oakland: New Harbinger Publications, Inc., 2014.

Spindler, Beth. *Yoga Therapy for Fear: Treating Anxiety, Depression and Rage with the Vagus Nerve and Other Techniques*. London: Singing Dragon, 2018.

Weintraub, Amy. *Yoga for Depression: A Compassionate Guide to Relieve Suffering Through Yoga*. New York: Broadway Books, 2004.

———. *Yoga Skills for Therapists: Effective Practices for Mood Management*. New York: W. W. Norton, 2012.

Yoga Service Council and Carol Horton, PhD. *Best Practices for Yoga with Veterans*. Vol. 2. Atlanta: YSC-Omega Publications, 2016.

Yoga, General Health, and Science

Broad, William J. *The Science of Yoga: The Risks and the Rewards*. New York: Simon and Schuster Paperbacks, 2012.

Costandi, Moheb. *Neuroplasticity: The MIT Press Essential Knowledge Series*. Cambridge, MA: MIT Press, 2016.

Khalsa, Sat Bir Singh, with Jodie Gould. *Your Brain on Yoga*. eBook. New York: Rosetta Books, 2012.

Khalsa, Sat Bir Singh, Lorenzo Cohen, Timothy McCall, and Shirley Telles. *Principles and Practice of Yoga in Health Care*. Edinburgh: Handspring Publishing, 2016.

General Yoga Practices (Poses and Breath Work)

Faulds, Richard. *Kripalu Yoga: A Guide to Practice On and Off the Mat*. New York: Bantam Books, 2006.

Freeman, Richard. *Yoga Breathing: Guided Instructions on the Art of Pranayama*. Audiobook. Louisville, CO: Sounds True, 2008.

Iyengar, B. K. S. *Light on Pranayama: The Yogic Art of Breathing*. New York: Crossroad, 1988.

———. *Light on Yoga: The Classic Guide to Yoga by the World's Foremost Author*. New York: HarperCollins, 2006.

———. *Yoga: The Path to Holistic Health*. New York: DK Publishing, 2001.

Lasater, Judith Hanson, PhD. *Relax and Renew: Restful Yoga for Stressful Times*, 2nd ed. Berkeley, CA: Rodmell Press, 2011.

———. *Restore and Rebalance: Yoga for Deep Relaxation*. Boulder, CO: Shambhala, 2017.

McCall, Timothy, MD. *Yoga as Medicine: The Yogic Prescription for Health and Healing*. New York: Bantam Dell, 2007.

Miller, Richard C., PhD. *Yoga Nidra: A Meditative Practice for Deep Relaxation and Healing*. Boulder, CO: Sounds True, 2010.

Rosen, Richard. *Pranayama Beyond the Fundamentals: An In-Depth Guide to Yogic Breathing*. Boston: Shambhala, 2006.

———. *The Yoga of Breath: A Step-by-Step Guide to Pranayama*. Boston: Shambhala, 2002.

Schiffman, Erich. *Yoga: The Spirit and Practice of Moving into Stillness*. New York: Pocket Books, 1996.

Sparrowe, Linda, and Patricia Walden. *The Woman's Book of Yoga & Health: A Life-long Guide to Wellness*. Boston: Shambhala, 2002.

Yoga Philosophy

Bryant, Edwin F., trans. *The Yoga Sutras of Patañjali: A New Edition, Translation, and Commentary*. New York: North Point Press, 2009.

Devi, Nischala Joy. *The Secret Power of Yoga: A Woman's Guide to the Heart and Spirit of the Yoga Sutras*. New York: Three Rivers Press, 2007.

Iyengar, B. K. S. *Light on Life: A Yoga Journey to Wholeness, Inner Peace, and Ultimate Freedom*. Emmaus, PA: Rodale Books, 2006.

———. *Light on the Yoga Sutras of Patañjali*. London: Thorsons, 1996.

Lasater, Judith Hanson, PhD. *Living Your Yoga: Finding the Spiritual in Everyday Life*. Berkeley, CA: Rodmell Press, 2000.

Miller, Barbara Stoler, trans. *The Bhagavad Gita: Krishna's Council in Time of War*. New York: Bantam Books, 1986.

Mitchell, Stephen, trans. *Bhagavad Gita: A New Translation*. New York: Harmony Books, 2000.

Roche, Loren, PhD. *The Radiance Sutras: 112 Tantra Yoga Teachings for Opening to the Divine in Everyday Life*. Marina Del Rey, CA: Syzygy Creations, 2008.

Shearer, Alistair, trans. *The Yoga Sutras of Patañjali*. New York: Bell Tower, 2002.

Stryker, Rod. *The Four Desires: Creating a Life of Purpose, Happiness, Prosperity and Freedom*. New York: Delacorte, 2011.

Other Holistic Practices for Mental Health

Brown, Richard, MD, and Patricia Gerbarg, MD. *The Healing Power of the Breath*. Boston: Shambhala, 2012.

Bullock, B. Grace. *Mindful Relationships: Seven Skills for Success—Integrating the Science of Mind, Body and Brain*. Edinburgh: Handspring Publishing, 2016.

Chodron, Pema. *Living Beautifully: With Uncertainty and Change*. Boston: Shambhala, 2012.

———. *When Things Fall Apart: Heart Advice for Difficult Times*. Boston: Shambhala, 2002.

Cope, Stephen. *The Great Work of Your Life: A Guide for the Journey to Your True Calling*. New York: Bantam, 2012.

Hanh, Thich Nhat. *The Art of Living: Peace and Freedom in the Here and Now*. San Francisco: HarperOne, 2017.

Kabat-Zinn, Jon. *Full Catastrophe Living: Using the Wisdom of Your Body and Mind to Face Stress, Pain, and Illness*. Rev. ed. New York: Bantam, 2013.

Naperstek, Belleruth. *Healing Trauma: Guided Imagery for Posttraumatic Stress*. Audiobook. Cleveland: Health Journeys, 2016.

———. *Peace Is Every Step: The Path of Mindfulness in Everyday Life*. New York: Bantam Books, 1992.

Tolle, Eckhart. *The Power of Now: A Guide to Spiritual Enlightenment*. Novato: New World Publishing, and Vancouver: Namaste Publishing, 2004.

———. *Stillness Speaks*. Novato: New World Publishing, and Vancouver: Namaste Publishing, 2003.

van der Kolk, Bessel A., MD. *The Body Keeps the Score: Brain, Mind, and Body in the Healing of Trauma*. New York: Penguin Books, 2015.

Scientific Journals

The following are scientific journals that publish new research on what's often called "complementary" medicine because it complements, or is helpful alongside, traditional medical treatments. In addition to perusing these journals, you can search for specific topics, like yoga and mental health, or look up specific studies like Dr. Streeter's research using the National Institutes of Health's "PubMed" catalog, which can be accessed online at https://www.ncbi.nlm.nih.gov/pubmed/.

Advances in Mind-Body Medicine
Complementary Therapies in Medicine
Evidence-Based Complementary and Alternative Medicine
International Journal of Yoga Therapy
Journal of Alternative and Complementary Medicine
Journal of Evidence-Based Complementary and Alternative Medicine

How to Find a Yoga Therapist

At the time of this writing, the International Association of Yoga Therapists (IAYT) is the largest internationally recognized certifying body for yoga therapists worldwide. In addition to awarding certifications (you will see the letters C-IAYT after the name of a yoga teacher who is certified), IAYT supports research and education through yoga therapy training programs. As of 2018, there were more than three thousand IAYT-certified yoga therapists; more than one thousand of these were in the United States. To find an IAYT-certified yoga therapist near you, visit https://www.iayt.org and click on "Find a Certified Yoga Therapist."

Not all yoga therapists are IAYT-certified, however. You can search for one in your area the same way you would seek out any holistic health professional. Ask questions about the practitioner's background, philosophy, and techniques. Ask for references from other students. Request a trial session. And most importantly, trust your instinct to discern whether a yoga therapist can support you in your healing journey.

NOTES

Preface

1. Weintraub, Amy, *Yoga for Depression: A Compassionate Guide to Relieve Suffering Through Yoga* (New York: Broadway Books, 2004), 9.

Chapter 1: The Journey Toward Becoming Whole Again

1. Gandhi, Mahatma, Quotes.net, https://www.quotes.net/quote/38145 (accessed September 26, 2018).

2. "Any Mood Disorder," National Institutes of Health, https://www.nimh.nih.gov/health/statistics/any-mood-disorder.shtml (accessed September 26, 2018).

3. "What Is Pranayama?" Integral Yoga Studio, http://www.integralyogastudio.com/pranayama.php (accessed September 26, 2018).

4. Avery, Helen, "Edwin Bryant: Why Read the Yoga Sutras," Wanderlust, https://wanderlust.com/journal/edwin-bryant-why-read-the-yoga-sutras/ (accessed September 26, 2018).

5. Streeter, Chris C., J. E. Jensen, R. M. Perlmutter, H. J. Cabral, H. Tian, D. B. Terhune, D. A. Ciraulo, and P. F. Renshaw, "Yoga Asana Sessions Increase Brain GABA Levels: A Pilot Study," *Journal of Alternative and Complementary Medicine* 13, no. 4 (2007): 419–426, https://www.ncbi.nlm.nih.gov/pubmed/17532734.

6. "2-Minute Neuroscience: GABA," Neuroscientifically Challenged, https://www.neuroscientificallychallenged.com/glossary/gaba/ (accessed September 26, 2018).

7. Carhart-Harris, R. L., and D. J. Nutt, "Serotonin and Brain Function: A Tale of Two Receptors," *Journal of Psychopharmacology* 31, no. 9 (2017): 1091–1120, https://www.ncbi.nlm.nih.gov/pmc/articles/PMC5606297/.

8. Iyengar, B. K. S., *Yoga: The Path to Holistic Health* (New York: DK Publishing, 2001), 365–369.

9. McCall, Timothy, MD, *Yoga as Medicine: The Yogic Prescription for Health and Healing* (New York: Bantam Dell, 2007), 261.

10. Broad, William J., *The Science of Yoga: The Risks and the Rewards* (New York: Simon & Schuster, 2012), xxx.

11. Brown, R. P., and P. L. Gerbarg, "Sudarshan Kriya Yogic Breathing in the Treatment of Stress, Anxiety, and Depression: Part II—Clinical Applications and Guidelines," *Journal of Alternative and Complementary Medicine* 11, no. 4 (2005): 711–717, https://www.ncbi.nlm.nih.gov/pubmed/16131297; Jindani, Farah, Nigel Turner, and Sat Bir S. Khalsa, "A Yoga Intervention for Posttraumatic Stress: A Preliminary Randomized Control Trial," *Evidence-based Complementary and Alternative Medicine* (2015): 351746, https://www.ncbi.nlm.nih.gov/pmc/articles/PMC4558444/; Gururaja, Derebail, Kaori Harano, Ikenaga Toyotake, and Haruo Kobayashi, "Effect of Yoga on Mental Health: Comparative Study Between Young and Senior Subjects in Japan," *International Journal of Yoga* 43, no. 1 (2011): 7–12, https://www.ncbi.nlm.nih.gov/pmc/articles/PMC3099103/.

12. Luscher, Bernhard, Qiuying Shen, and Nadia Sahir, "The GABAergic Deficit Hypothesis of Major Depressive Disorder," *Molecular Psychiatry* 16, no. 4 (2010): 383–406, https://www.ncbi.nlm.nih.gov/pmc/articles/PMC3412149/.

13. Streeter, Chris C., T. H. Whitfield, L. Owen, T. Rein, S. K. Karri, A. Yakhind, R. Perlmutter, A. Prescot, P. F. Renshaw, D. A. Ciraulo, and J. E. Jensen, "Effects of Yoga Versus Walking on Mood, Anxiety, and Brain GABA Levels: A Randomized Controlled MRS Study," *Journal of Alternative and Complementary Medicine* 16, no. 11 (2010): 1145–1152, https://www.ncbi.nlm.nih.gov/pubmed/20722471.

14. Gauvin, L., and W. J. Rejeski, "The Exercise-Induced Feeling Inventory: Development and Initial Validation," *Journal of Sport and Exercise Psychology* 15, no. 4 (1993): 403–423; Spielberger, C. D., *State-Trait Anxiety Inventory: Bibliography*, 2nd ed. (Palo Alto: Consulting Psychologists Press, 1989).

15. Streeter Chris C., P. L. Gerbarg, R. B. Saper, D. A. Ciraulo, and R. P. Brown, "Effects of Yoga on the Autonomic Nervous System, Gamma-Aminobutryic-Acid, and Allostatis in Epilepsy, Depression, and Posttraumatic Stress Disorder," *Medical Hypotheses* 78, no. 5 (2012): 571–579, https://www.ncbi.nlm.nih.gov/pubmed/22365651.

16. Streeter et al., "Effects of Yoga Versus Walking."

17. "How Does the Nervous System Work?" National Center for Biotechnology Information, https://www.ncbi.nlm.nih.gov/books/NBK279390/ (accessed February 13, 2019).

18. Porges, Stephen W., "Social Engagement and Attachment: A Phylogenetic Perspective," *New York Academy of Sciences* 1008 (2003): 34, http://www.somatic practice.net/trainings/touch_skills/resources/articles/polyvagal/Porges-2003-Social _Engagement_and_Attachment.pdf.

19. Streeter et al., "Effects of Yoga on the Autonomic Nervous System."

20. Streeter et al., "Yoga Asana Sessions Increase Brain GABA Levels."

21. Ibid.

22. Streeter, Chris C., P. L. Gerbarg, T. H. Whitfield, L. Owen, J. Johnson, M. M. Silveri, M. Gensler, C. L. Faulkner, C. Mann, M. Wixted, A. M. Hernon, M. B. Nyer, E. R. Brown, and J. E. Jensen, "Treatment of Major Depressive Disorder with Iyengar Yoga and Coherent Breathing: A Randomized Controlled Dosing Study," *Journal of Alternative and Complementary Medicine* 23, no. 3 (2017): 201–207, https://www.ncbi .nlm.nih.gov/pubmed/28296480.

23. Brown, Richard, MD, and Patricia Gerbarg, MD, *The Healing Power of the Breath* (Boston: Shambhala, 2012).

24. Beck, A. T., C. H. Ward, M. Mendelson, J. Mock, and J. Erbaugh, "An Inventory for Measuring Depression," *Archives of General Psychiatry* 4 (1961): 561–571.

25. "Beck Depression Inventory II: How to Use," PsychCongress, https://www .psychcongress.com/saundras-corner/scales-screenersdepression/beck-depression -inventory-ii-bdi-ii (accessed September 26, 2018).

26. Streeter, Chris C., P. L. Gerbarg, T. H. Whitfield, L. Owen, J. Johnson, M. M. Silveri, M. Gensler, C. L. Faulkner, C. Mann, M. Wixted, A. M. Hernon, M. B. Nyer, E. R. Brown, and J. E. Jensen, "Treatment of Major Depressive Disorder with Iyengar Yoga and Coherent Breathing: A Randomized Controlled Dosing Study," *Journal of Alternative and Complementary Medicine* 23, no. 3 (2017): 201–207, https://www.ncbi .nlm.nih.gov/pubmed/28296480.

27. MacMillan, Amanda, "It's Official: Yoga Helps Depression," *Time*, http://time .com/4695558/yoga-breathing-depression/ (accessed September 26, 2018).

28. Streeter et al., "Treatment of Major Depressive Disorder with Iyengar Yoga and Coherent Breathing."

29. Streeter et al., "Effects of Yoga Versus Walking."

30. Two studies support the idea that a range of one to five yoga classes per week can be helpful for those with depression: H. Cramer et al., "A Systematic Review of Yoga for Major Depressive Disorder," *Journal of Affective Disorders* 213 (2017): 70–77, https://www.ncbi.nlm.nih.gov/pubmed/28192737; and L. A. Uebelacker et al., "Adjunctive Yoga v. Health Education for Persistent Major Depression: A Randomized

Controlled Trial," *Psychological Medicine* 47, no. 12 (2017): 2130–2142, https://www
.ncbi.nlm.nih.gov/pubmed/28382883.

31. Porges, Stephen W., PhD, *The Polyvagal Theory: Neurophysiological Foundations of Emotions, Attachment, Communication, and Self-Regulation* (New York: W. W. Norton, 2011).

32. Seymour, Tom, "Everything You Need to Know About the Vagus Nerve," MedicaNewsToday, https://www.medicalnewstoday.com/articles/318128.php (accessed September 26, 2018).

33. Streeter et al., "Effects of Yoga on the Autonomic Nervous System."

34. Porges, Stephen W., "The Polyvagal Theory: Phylogenetic Substrates of a Social Nervous System," *International Journal of Psychopsysiology* 42 (2001): 123–146, http://www.terapiacognitiva.eu/cpc/dwl/polivagale/polyvagal_theory.pdf.

35. Streeter et al., "Effects of Yoga on the Autonomic Nervous System."

36. Porges, Stephen W., "Polyvagal Theory: How Your Body Makes the Decision," YouTube, https://www.youtube.com/watch?v=ivLEAlhBHPM (accessed June 13, 2019).

37. Porges, Stephen W., "Social Engagement and Attachment: A Phylogenetic Perspective," *New York Academy of Sciences* 1008 (2003): 34, http://www.somatic practice.net/trainings/touch_skills/resources/articles/polyvagal/Porges-2003-Social _Engagement_and_Attachment.pdf.

38. Porges, Stephen W., "The Polyvagal Theory," YouTube, https://www.youtube .com/watch?v=8tz146HQotY (accessed September 26, 2018).

39. Chen, Jenny, "Why Depression Needs a New Definition," *The Atlantic*, https://www.theatlantic.com/health/archive/2015/08/why-depression-needs-a-new -definition/399902/ (accessed September 26, 2018).

40. To highlight the speed at which this understanding is progressing, it was just in 2007 that Dr. Timothy McCall, in his book *Yoga as Medicine* (New York: Bantam Dell, 2007), 263, described an "increasing" view among doctors of "depression as a biochemical problem, related to abnormal levels of neurotransmitters like serotonin, norepinephrine, and dopamine in the brain." Today, other brain mechanisms, including new cell growth, are "increasingly" viewed as promising avenues for determining the causes of and best treatment for depression.

41. Costandi, Moheb, *Neuroplasticity: The MIT Press Essential Knowledge Series* (Cambridge, MA: MIT Press, 2016), 11.

42. Kupfer, David J., MD, "Depression and the New DSM-5 Classification," Medicographia, https://www.medicographia.com/2015/06/depression-and -the-new-dsm-5-classification/ (accessed September 26, 2018); "Definitions: Major

Depression," National Institute of Mental Health, https://www.nimh.nih.gov/health
/statistics/major-depression.shtml (accessed February 13, 2019).

43. "Definitions: Any Anxiety Disorder," National Institute of Mental Health,
https://www.nimh.nih.gov/health/statistics/any-anxiety-disorder.shtml (accessed February 13, 2019).

44. Paul, S. M.,"Anxiety and Depression: A Common Neurobiological Sub-
strate?" *Journal of Clinical Psychology* 49, Supplement (October 1988): 13–16, https://
www.ncbi.nlm.nih.gov/pubmed/2844736.

45. "Depression DSM-5 Diagnostic Criteria," PsyCom, https://www.psycom.net
/depression-definition-dsm-5-diagnostic-criteria/#dsm-5diagnosticcriteria (accessed
February 13, 2019).

46. Rowling, J. K., *Harry Potter and the Sorcerer's Stone* (New York: Arthur A.
Levine Books, 1997), 298.

47. Khalsa, Guruchan Singh, "Happiness Is Your Birthright," 3HO: Healthy,
Happy, Holy Organization, https://www.3ho.org/homepage-tabs/happiness-your
-birthright (accessed September 26, 2018).

Chapter 2: How Yoga Can Support Your Healing Journey

1. Weintraub, Amy, *Yoga for Depression: A Compassionate Guide to Relieve Suffering Through Yoga* (New York: Broadway Books, 2004), 80.

2. Khalsa, Guruchan Singh, "Happiness Is Your Birthright," 3HO: Healthy,
Happy, Holy Organization, https://www.3ho.org/homepage-tabs/happiness-your
-birthright (accessed September 26, 2018).

3. Bryant, Edwin F., *The Yoga Sutras of Patañjali: A New Edition, Translation, and
Commentary* (New York: North Point Press, 2009), 169.

4. Iyengar, B. K. S., *Light on the Yoga Sutras of Patañjali* (New Delhi: HarperCollins
Publishers, 1993), 102.

5. Weintraub, *Yoga for Depression*, 75.

6. Bryant, *The Yoga Sutras of Patañjali*, 572–574; and Rolf Sovik, *The Gunas: Nature's Three Fundamental Forces*, Yoga International, https://yogainternational.com
/article/view/the-gunas-natures-three-fundamental-forces (accessed February 13, 2019).

7. For a more detailed discussion of *rajasic* and *tamasic* depression, see Timothy
McCall, MD, *Yoga as Medicine: The Yogic Prescription for Health and Healing* (New
York: Bantam Books, 2007), 267.

8. The Sufi mystic poet Rumi captures an image similar to the emotional dinner
party I'm describing in his poem "The Guest House." The poem begins, "This being

human is a guest house. / Every morning a new arrival. / A joy, a depression, a mean-ness, / some momentary awareness comes / as an unexpected visitor." "The Guest House," in *The Essential Rumi: New Expanded Edition*, translated by Coleman Barks (San Francisco: Harper San Francisco, 2004), 109.

9. Iyengar, *Light on the Yoga Sutras of Patañjali*, 129.

10. Shearer, Alistair, *The Yoga Sutras of Patañjali* (New York: Bell Tower, 1982), 90.

11. For a more comprehensive list, visit the Center for Nonviolent Commu-nication's "Feelings Inventory," https://www.cnvc.org/sites/default/files/feelings _inventory_0.pdf, or see the work of Barbara Frederickson, who runs the Positive Emotions and Psychophysiology Laboratory (PEP Lab) at the University of North Carolina at Chapel Hill. Her work explores the myriad variations of emotional life, focusing especially on positive emotions. See https://www.positivityratio.com/.

12. For a discussion of the term, see Iyengar, *Light on the Yoga Sutras of Patañjali*, 137. For definitions of the Sanskrit words, see "Pratipaksha," SpokenSanskrit.org, http://spokensanskrit.org/index.php?mode=3&script=hk&tran_input=pratipaksha &direct=au (accessed October 5, 2018); and "Bhavana," SpokenSanskrit.org, http:// spokensanskrit.org/index.php?mode=3&script=hk&tran_input=bhavana&direct=au (accessed October 5, 2018).

Chapter 3: The Life Force in Your Body

1. Feuerstein, Georg, PhD, *The Shambhala Encyclopedia of Yoga* (Boston: Sham-bhala, 1997), 194.

2. Ibid., 127.

3. "Pingala," Yogapedia, https://www.yogapedia.com/definition/6180/pingala (ac-cessed October 5, 2018).

4. Feuerstein, Georg, PhD, and Larry Payne, PhD, *Yoga for Dummies* (Foster City CA: IDG Books Worldwide, 1999), 293.

5. Bailey, James, "Discover the Ida and Pingala Nadis," YogaJournal, https://www .yogajournal.com/yoga-101/balancing-act-2 (accessed October 5, 2018).

6. Feuerstein and Payne, *Yoga for Dummies*, 294.

7. LePage, Joseph and Lillian, *Yoga Teachers' Toolbox* (Santa Rosa, CA: Integra-tive Yoga Therapy, 2005), 3.

8. Saradananda, Swami, *Mudras for Modern Life* (London: Watkins Media Lim-ited, 2015), 138 and 62.

Chapter 4: Getting Ready for Your Yoga Practice

1. Streeter, Chris C., P. L. Gerbarg, T. H. Whitfield, L. Owen, J. Johnson, M. M. Silveri, M. Gensler, C. L. Faulkner, C. Mann, M. Wixted, A. M. Hernon, M. B. Nyer, E. R. Brown, and J. E. Jensen, "Treatment of Major Depressive Disorder with Iyengar Yoga and Coherent Breathing: A Randomized Controlled Dosing Study," *Journal of Alternative and Complementary Medicine* 23, no. 3 (2017): 201–207, https://www.ncbi .nlm.nih.gov/pubmed/28296480.

2. Walden, Patricia, with Jarvis Chen, ScD, *Yoga for Emotional Healing* (self-published, 2009), 10–19. See also B. K. S. Iyengar, *Yoga: The Path to Holistic Health* (New York: DK Publishing, 2001), 365–369.

3. Walden and Chen, *Yoga for Emotional Healing*, 10.

4. Brown, Richard P., MD, and Patricia L. Gerbarg, MD, *The Healing Power of the Breath* (Boston: Shambhala, 2012), 12.

5. This study's findings suggest that consistent yoga practice "tunes the brain" toward a parasympathetic-dominant state: Villemure, Chantal, Marta Ceko, Valerie A. Cotton, and M. Catherine Bushness, "Neuroprotective Effects of Yoga Practice: Age-, Experience-, and Frequency-Dependent Plasticity," *Frontiers in Human Neuroscience* 9 (2015): 281, https://www.ncbi.nlm.nih.gov/pmc/articles/PMC4428135/.

6. Kempton, Sally, "Take the Plunge!" Sally Kempton, https://www.sallykempton .com/resources/articles/take-the-plunge/ (accessed October 5, 2018).

7. McCall, Timothy, MD, *Yoga as Medicine: The Yogic Prescription for Health and Healing* (New York: Random House, 2007), 261.

8. Walden and Chen, *Yoga for Emotional Healing*, 10.

9. Sarananda, Swami, *Mudras for Modern Life* (London: Watkins, 2015), 138.

10. McCall, *Yoga as Medicine*, 266.

11. Iyengar, B. K. S., *Yoga: The Path to Holistic Health* (New York: DK Publishing, 2001), 183, 365–369.

12. Ibid., 234.

13. Feuerstein, Georg, PhD, and Larry Payne, PhD, *Yoga for Dummies* (Foster City, CA: IDG Books Worldwide, 1999), 166.

14. "Deep Relaxation Boosts Health at a Genetic Level," Natural Health News, https://www.naturalhealthnews.uk/mind-body/2013/05/deep-relaxation-boosts -health-at-a-genetic-level/ (accessed October 5, 2018).

15. Ibid.

16. Elliott, Stephen, with Dee Edmonson, RN, *The New Science of Breath,*

Coherent Breathing for Autonomic Nervous System Balance, Health, and Well-Being, 2nd ed. (Allen, TX: Coherence Press, 2006), 31.

17. Brown and Gerbarg, *The Healing Power of the Breath*, 20–21.

Chapter 5: Center

1. "Center," Merriam-Webster, https://www.merriam-webster.com/dictionary/center (accessed November 27, 2018).

2. Hanh, Thich Nhat, "Transforming Feelings," Living Life Fully, http://www.livinglifefully.com/flo/flobetransformingfeelings.htm (accessed September 27, 2018).

3. Shearer, Alistair, *The Yoga Sutras of Patañjali* (New York: Bell Tower, 1982), 115.

4. Iyengar, B. K. S., *Light on the Yoga Sutras of Patañjali* (New Delhi: HarperCollins, 1993), 151.

5. "Vrska," SpokenSanskrit.org, http://spokensanskrit.org/index.php?mode=3&script=hk&tran_input=vrksa&direct=au (accessed October 7, 2018).

6. van der Kolk, Bessel, MD, *The Body Keeps the Score: Brain, Mind, and Body in the Healing of Trauma* (New York: Penguin Books, 2014), 275.

7. Streeter, Chris C., P. L. Gerbarg, R. B. Saper, D. A. Ciraulo, and R. P. Brown, "Effects of Yoga on the Autonomic Nervous System, Gamma-Aminobutryic-Acid, and Allostatis in Epilepsy, Depression, and Posttraumatic Stress Disorder," *Medical Hypotheses* 78, no. 5 (2012): 571–579, https://www.ncbi.nlm.nih.gov/pubmed/22365651.

8. Iyengar, *Light on the Yoga Sutras of Patañjali*, 159.

9. Roche, Lorin, PhD, *The Radiance Sutras* (Marina del Rey, CA: Syzygy Creations, 2008), 111.

10. McGreevey, Sue, "Eight Weeks to a Better Brain," Harvard University, http://news.harvard.edu/gazette/story/2011/01/eight-weeks-to-a-better-brain/ (accessed September 27, 2018).

11. "Anahata," SpokenSanskrit.org, http://spokensanskrit.org/index.php?mode=3&script=hk&tran_input=anahata&direct=au (accessed October 7, 2018).

12. Roche, *The Radiance Sutras*, 111.

13. Devi, Nischala Joy, *The Secret Power of Yoga: A Woman's Guide to the Heart and Spirit of the Yoga Sutras* (New York: Three Rivers Press, 2007), 289.

Chapter 6: Empower

1. Mitchell, Stephen, *Bhagavad Gita: A New Translation* (New York: Harmony Books, 2000), 51.
2. Ibid., 65.
3. Ibid., 53.
4. Ibid., 134.

Chapter 7: Energize

1. "Prana," Yogapedia, https://www.yogapedia.com/definition/5154/prana (accessed February 13, 2019).
2. Feuerstein, Georg, *The Shambhala Encyclopedia of Yoga* (Boston: Shambhala, 1997), 157.
3. McCall, Timothy, MD, *Yoga as Medicine: The Yogic Prescription for Health and Healing* (New York: Bantam Dell, 2007), 267.
4. Sovik, Rolf, *The Gunas: Nature's Three Fundamental Forces*, Yoga International, https://yogainternational.com/article/view/the-gunas-natures-three-fundamental -forces (accessed February 13, 2019).
5. Koukopoulos, A., "Agitated Depression as a Mixed State and the Problem of Melancholia," *Psychiatric Clinics of North America* 2022, no. 203, September 1, 1999, 547–564, https://www.ncbi.nlm.nih.gov/pubmed/10550855.
6. "Abhaya Mudra," Yogapedia, https://yogapedia.com/definition/7615/abhaya -mudra (accessed October 8, 2018).

Chapter 8: Calm

1. "Ellen DeGeneres Quotes," BrainyQuote, https://www.brainyquote.com /quotes/ellen_degeneres_451786 (accessed September 27, 2018).
2. "Shanti," Yogapedia, https://www.yogapedia.com/definition/5032/shanti (accessed September 27, 2018).
3. Dankosky, John, and William Broad, "The Science of Yoga: The Risks and the Rewards," interview, National Public Radio, https://www.npr .org/2012/02/10/146697650/the-science-of-yoga-the-risks-and-the-rewards (accessed September 27, 2018).
4. "The Stress/Threat Response Cycle," Discovery Healing, https://discovery healing.com/the-stressthreat-response-cycle/ (accessed September 27, 2018).

5. Streeter, Chris C., P. L. Gerberg, R. B. Saper, D. A. Ciraulo, and R. P. Brown, "Effects of Yoga on the Autonomic Nervous System, Gamma-Aminobutryic-Acid, and Allostatis in Epilepsy, Depression, and Posttraumatic Stress Disorder," *Medical Hypotheses* 78, no. 5 (2012): 571–579, https://www.ncbi.nlm.nih.gov/pubmed/2236 5651.

6. Iyengar, B. K. S., John Evans, and Douglas Abrams, *Light on Life: The Yoga Journey to Wholeness, Inner Peace, and Ultimate Freedom* (New York: Rodale, 2005), 107.

7. van der Kolk, Bessel, "Bessel van der Kolk on Interoception and Yoga," YouTube, https://www.youtube.com/watch?v=_pxp9958_Eo (accessed September 27, 2018).

8. Nguyen, Anh-Huong, and Thich Nhat Hanh, *Walking Meditation* (Boulder, CO: Sounds True, 2006), 22.

Chapter 9: Balance

1. Sovik, Rolf, "The Gunas: Nature's Three Fundamental Forces," YogaInternational, https://yogainternational.com/article/view/the-gunas-natures-three -fundamental-forces (accessed February 13, 2019).

2. Forbes, Bo, *Yoga for Emotional Balance: Simple Practices to Help Relieve Anxiety and Depression* (Boston: Shambhala, 2011), 6.

3. Shearer, Alastair, *The Yoga Sutras of Patañjali* (New York: Bell Tower, 1982), 111.

4. "Viveka," SpokenSanskrit.org, http://spokensanskrit.org/index.php?mode =3&script=hk&tran_input=viveka&direct=au (accessed February 13, 2019).

5. Shearer, *The Yoga Sutras of Patañjali*, 115–116.

6. "Samasthiti," Yogapedia, https://www.yogapedia.com/definition/6429 /samasthiti (accessed February 13, 2019).

7. Walden, Patricia, with Jarvis Chen, ScD, *Yoga for Emotional Healing* (self-published, 2009), 9.

Chapter 10: Looking Ahead with Hope and Confidence

1. Brown, Brené, *I Thought It Was Just Me: Women Reclaiming Power and Courage in a Culture of Shame* (New York: Gotham, 2007), xxiii.

2. You can find out more about ecopsychology at https://www.ecopsychology .org, or subscribe to *Ecopsychology*, the only peer-reviewed scientific journal focused

exclusively on the connection between psychology, mental health, and ecology, at https://home.liebertpub.com/publications/ecopsychology/300.

3. Song, C., H. Ikei, M. Igarashi, M. Takagaki, and Y. Miyazaki, "Physiological and Psychological Effects of a Walk in Urban Parks in Fall," *International Journal of Environmental Research and Public Health* 12, no. 11 (2015): 14216–14228, https://www.ncbi.nlm.nih.gov/pmc/articles/PMC4661642/.

4. van Praag, C., S. Garfinkel, O. Sparasci, A. Mees, A. Philippides, M. Ware, C. Ottaviani, and H. Critchley, "Mind-Wandering and Alterations to Default Mode Network Connectivity When Listening to Naturalistic Versus Artificial Sounds," *Scientific Reports* 7 (2017): 45273, https://www.ncbi.nlm.nih.gov/pmc/articles/PMC5366899/.

5. Tolle, Eckhart, *Stillness Speaks* (San Francisco: New World Library, 2003), 5.

6. Brown, Richard, MD, and Patricia Gerbarg, MD, *The Healing Power of the Breath* (Boston: Shambhala, 2012), 134.

7. "How Much Sleep Do I Need?" Centers for Disease Control and Prevention, https://www.cdc.gov/sleep/about_sleep/how_much_sleep.html (accessed October 29, 2018).

8. "Yogi Bhajan Quotes on Community," Health, Happy, Holy Organization, https://www.3ho.org/yogi-bhajan-quotes-community (accessed October 29, 2018).

9. Kempton, Sally, "Take the Plunge!" Sally Kempton, https://www.sallykempton.com/resources/articles/take-the-plunge/ (accessed October 5, 2018).

10. Philosophico Literary Research Department of Kaivalyadhama S. M. Y. M. Samiti, Lonavla, India, *Yoga Kosha* (New Delhi: Model Press, 1991), 323.

INDEX

ida (channel of comfort), 28
inhibitory neurotransmitters, 5
inner strength. *See* empowerment/
 empowering practice
intellectual body (*vijnanamaya kosha*), 95
inversions, 37, 49–50
Inverted Pose, 49
 Balancing, 143–144
 Calming, 124–125
 Centering, 70–72
 Empowering, 88–90
 Energizing, 106
Iyengar, B. K. S., 6, 40, 114
Iyengar yoga, 6, 37

Kempton, Sally, 40, 156
koshas (bodies), 95

life force (*prana*), 28, 94

magnetic resonance spectroscopy (MRS), 8
Major Depressive Disorder (MDD)
 criteria for, 16
 prevalence of, 15
Manipura chakra (navel chakra), 29, 30
manomaya kosha (thought body), 95
Marichi's Twist I, 104–105
mat, 34
meditation, 156–157
mental health, yoga's impact on, 5–7
mind-body relationship, 4–5, 19
mood disorders, prevalence of, 4
Mountain Pose, 42, 46
mudras (hand positions), 31
Muladhara chakra (root chakra), 29, 30
myelin, 13–14

nadis (energetic pathways), 28, 29
National Center for Complementary and
 Integrative Health, 7
National Institutes of Health, 4, 7, 15
nature, 150–151
navel chakra (*Manipura chakra*), 29, 30
neuroplasticity, 15, 26

Ocean Breath
 Centering Pose with, 38–40
 Cross-Legged Seated Pose with, 60–62,
 80–81, 99–100, 116–117, 135–136
 daily practice of, 151–152
 Deep Relaxation with, 50–51, 72–74,
 90–91, 107–108, 126–127, 146–148
 polyvagal theory and, 13
 sleep and, 153
one-pointedness, 58

parasympathetic nervous system (PNS),
 9–10, 13, 38, 61, 113
physical alignment–based yoga system, 6
physical body (*annamaya kosha*), 95
pingala (solar current), 28
Plow Pose and Shoulder Stand, 144–146
polyvagal theory, 10, 13–14
Porges, Stephen, 13–14
poses
 Balancing Inverted Pose, 143–144
 Boat Pose, 136–137
 Bridge Pose, 103–104
 Calming Inverted Pose, 124–125
 Centering Inverted Pose, 70–72
 Centering Pose with Ocean Breath,
 38
 Child's Pose, 67–68, 122–123
 Cobra Pose, 44
 Cross-Legged Seated Pose with Ocean
 Breath, 60–62, 80–81, 99–100,
 116–117, 135–136
 Downward Facing Dog Pose, 43, 45
 Empowering Inverted Pose, 88–90
 Energizing Inverted Pose, 106
 Four Limb Staff Pose, 44
 Head-to-Knee Pose, 87–88
 Hero's Pose with Cow-Face Arms,
 100–101
 Hero's Pose with Upward Bound
 Knuckle Pose, 81–82
 High Plank Pose, 44
 Inverted Pose, 49
 Mountain Pose, 42, 46